Diuretic Agents

Edward J. Cragoe, Jr., EDITOR

Merck Sharp and Dohme Research Laboratories

Based on a symposium

sponsored by the ACS

Division of Medicinal

Chemistry at the 174th

Meeting of the American

Chemical Society, Chicago,

Illinois, August 29, 1977.

ACS SYMPOSIUM SERIES 83

AMERICAN CHEMICAL SOCIETY

WASHINGTON, D. C.   1978

Library of Congress CIP Data

Diuretic agents.
   (ACS symposium series; 83 ISSN 0097-6156)

   Includes bibliographies and index.

   1. Diuretics and diuresis—Congresses. 2. Chemistry,
Pharmaceutical—Congresses.
   I. Cragoe, Edward J. II. American Chemical Society.
Division of Medicinal Chemistry. III. Series: American
Chemical Society. ACS symposium series: 83.

RS431.D58D58   615'.761   78-23405
ISBN 0-8412-0464-0   ASCMC 8   83 1–238 1978

Copyright © 1978

American Chemical Society

ACS Symposium Series

Robert F. Gould, *Editor*

FOREWORD

The ACS SYMPOSIUM SERIES was founded in 1974 to provide a medium for publishing symposia quickly in book form. The format of the SERIES parallels that of the continuing ADVANCES IN CHEMISTRY SERIES except that in order to save time the papers are not typeset but are reproduced as they are submitted by the authors in camera-ready form. As a further means of saving time, the papers are not edited or reviewed except by the symposium chairman, who becomes editor of the book. Papers published in the ACS SYMPOSIUM SERIES are original contributions not published elsewhere in whole or major part and include reports of research as well as reviews since symposia may embrace both types of presentation.

CONTENTS

PREFACE

Some scientists believe that man is a brain surrounded by cells of secondary significance while others are persuaded that the heart takes preeminence. Of course, neither is correct; man consists of two magnificent organs called kidneys which are imbedded in tissues of lesser importance. Seriously, the kidney provides a pervasive, homeostatic regulation of the entire internal environment of the body; more specifically, kidney function modulates electrolyte and fluid balances, the economy of nutrients and drugs, and the formation and elimination of metabolites. Because the kidney is involved either directly or indirectly with nearly every cellular process, the ability of this organ to function properly under conditions of stress, age, or disease becomes progressively more important and, ultimately often becomes the limiting factor in the survival of the body itself. Since water and electrolyte are the major constituents of terrestrial life, organs that control their transport are of vital importance.

Since the beginning of modern medicine, the discovery and use of drugs which control renal function have been a major goal. Only a small portion of what may be considered to be the full potential of this field has been realized. Future achievements in this area are certain to come, albeit with many birth pangs.

The first drugs developed for the control of renal function were the diuretics which also were among the first synthetic agents to be introduced into medicine. Although modern diuretic therapy is not yet three decades old, a series of prominent milestones mark its history, and this history is still being made. The outstanding and continuing record of the development of novel diuretic agents has greatly enhanced the progress of the basic science relating to kidney function. This fundamental knowledge has, in turn, permitted the discovery of even more unique diuretics. Most importantly, these drugs are as safe and sophisticated as any that are in our present medical armamentarium.

Mercurial agents constituted the first chemical class of the synthetic diuretics, and these drugs possessed many commendable attributes, including a good electrolyte excretion profile, high potency, and uricosuric activity. Within a few years, the carbonic anhydrase inhibitors were discovered which provided a more practical therapy. The advent of the thiazides opened the door to a deluge of structurally and functionally related sulfonamide diuretics. The loop diuretics, as represented by furosemide and ethacrynic acid, constituted the next major breakthrough. Finally, the antikaliuretic saluretics, i.e., aldactone, triamterene, and amiloride, entered the arena.

During their short history in medicine, the demand for and the use of diuretics has increased dramatically. It is estimated that the world-wide use of diuretics involved ten billion patient days in 1977 at a cost of $765 million. If the use of diuretics increases at its present rate, it will double within the next five or six years. Interestingly, the use of diuretics for the treatment of hypertension is growing at a faster rate than that for edema. Another obvious trend is the shift away from the use of potassium-losing diuretics to that of the antikaliuretic diuretics, either alone or in combination.

Research activity and the resultant major "breakthroughs" in the diuretic field have occurred sporadically and, if the current signs are valid, we are in the midst of a new phase of intense research activity. Although a number of safe and effective diuretics are available, they each have inherent deficiencies which impart to them a significant obsolescence liability. The most prevalent problems include hypokalemia, hyperglycemia, and hyperuricemia. In addition, most diuretics belong to a very small group of chemical or structural classes. As a result, they have similar mechanisms of action and side effects. The diuretics of the future must be structurally novel and mechanistically unique and, more importantly, they must obviate many of the side effects that are characteristic of the agents currently in use.

The rapid advances that have been made in the sciences which are basic to the understanding of water and electrolyte transport have permitted a more sophisticated approach to the design of new diuretics. It also has allowed the early examination of new leads for their site and mechanism of action. Progress in the biochemistry of electrolyte transport has been noteworthy in recent years, especially in regard to the role of renal hormones. Likewise, advances in micropuncture and a variety of other techniques have provided tools which are useful for the routine evaluation and recognition of truly novel renal agents.

It has been 15 years since deStevens' classic monograph (1) on the medicinal chemistry of diuretics appeared. Therefore, a symposium (2) was organized which was designed to review the progress that had occurred in the intervening years. Since the symposium was limited to only a one-half-day session, it was not possible to include reports from every institution where major discoveries had been made. The interest generated by the symposium suggested that the papers be published. In order to present a more complete picture of the innovative research in this field, both from the standpoint of the basic science and of the practical agents available at the clinical level, four more papers were added to those of the original symposium.

Since the main purpose of this monograph was to describe the recent advances in the medicinal chemistry of diuretics, the emphasis was placed on the fundamental contributions of the medicinal chemists, i.e., drug design and structure–activity relationships. The authors of this monograph and the institutions that they represent have made particularly noteworthy contributions to renal research and many of them have been associated with a long history of outstanding work.

On the academic side, it seemed only appropriate to include the recent work on the prostaglandin and kallikrein–kinin systems. The role of these renal hormones is extremely complex and currently in a state of refinement, but it is of such importance that it demands consideration by all scientists involved in renal research.

Examination of the history and current status of the diuretic field not only permits but encourages extrapolation into the future. Such extrapolation suggests that significant diuretics which will emerge will have novel structures, unique mechanisms, and new sites of action. More importantly, new types of renal agents will be discovered which will provide for the prophylaxis and treatment of renal disorders where no drug is currently available.

Acknowledgments—Many people have contributed to the planning and programming of the diuretic symposium and to the writing of this book. The authors of each paper have been extremely cooperative and helpful, not only in providing their contribution, but in integrating their unit into the whole. Much editorial assistance and advice were provided by E. H. Blaine, M. G. Bock, S. J. deSolms, R. L. Smith, A. K. Willard, and O. W. Woltersdorf, Jr. I am indebted to Florence Berg for checking and editing the bibliographies of many of the manuscripts.

I am most grateful to my secretary, C. F. Slobodzian, for the exceptional job she did in typing and proofreading each draft of many of these manuscripts and of the final draft of most of the others. She also provided invaluable assistance in the voluminous correspondence required in organizing the symposium and writing the book.

Literature Cited—

1. deStevens, G., "Medicinal Chemistry, a Series of Monographs, Vol. 1, Diuretics: Chemistry and Pharmacology," Academic, New York, 1963.
2. *National Meeting of the American Chemical Society, 174th,* Symposium on Diuretic Agents, Medicinal Chemistry papers 1–7, 1977.

Merck Sharp and Dohme Research   EDWARD J. CRAGOE, JR.
   Laboratories
West Point, Pennsylvania
August 21, 1978

Prostaglandins and Renal Function: Implications for the Activity of Diuretic Agents

J. C. McGIFF and P. Y-K WONG

Department of Pharmacology and Department of Medicine, University of Tennessee Center for the Health Sciences, Memphis, TN 38163

Prostaglandins are primarily local or tissue hormones which act at or near their sites of synthesis and are synthesized on demand as they are not stored (1). In the kidney, as in other tissues, prostaglandins serve primarily a defensive function, although they may contribute to the maintenance of renal function under physiological conditions. Furosemide, ethacrynic acid and bumetanide, the most potent of the diuretic agents, can cause a precipitous decline in renal function, particularly in the sodium depleted subject; a prostaglandin response evoked in response to the "loop diuretic" may maintain renal function in the face of this challenge (2). The capacity of the kidney to respond to a stimulus which depresses renal function by increasing prostaglandin synthesis was first shown during administration of a vasoconstrictor agent such as angiotensin or norepinephrine (3). Release of prostaglandins coincided with restoration of renal blood flow and urine flow despite continued administration of either angiotensin II or norepinephrine.

STRESS EVOKED RENAL PROSTAGLANDIN RESPONSE

A prostaglandin mechanism seems important to the regulation of the renal circulation when the latter is compromised by an acute insult or chronic disease. For example, activation of the renin-angiotensin system by either hemorrhage (4), laparotomy (5) or a "loop diuretic" can increase synthesis of prostaglandins by the kidney; the concentration of PGE_2 in renal venous blood increased by as much as fifteen-fold during surgical stress and was closely correlated with the level of plasma renin activity (5). Thus, under acute stress the activities of the renin-angiotensin and prostaglandin systems within the kidney appear to be coupled. The contribution of a prostaglandin mechanism to the support of the renal circulation in the acutely stressed dog may be uncovered by administration of indomethacin, an inhibitor of prostaglandin synthesis (5). A large reduction in renal blood flow occurred rapidly in response to indomethacin, despite an

attendant increase in renal perfusion pressure. There was a
simultaneous decline in renal efflux of PGE_2 which was propor-
tional to the reduction in renal blood flow. This study demonstrated that in the animal subjected to acute stress, the renal
circulation was supported by a major prostaglandin component,
withdrawal of which resulted in decreased renal blood flow,
particularly that fraction to the inner cortex and medulla (7).

PROSTAGLANDIN RELATED EFFECTS ON RENAL BLOOD FLOW

The pattern of distribution of blood flow within the kidney
may affect salt and water excretion; for example, increased blood
flow to the medulla can lower the tonicity of the medullary
interstitium and, thereby, diminish the capacity to concentrate
urine, resulting in increased water excretion. Changes in
prostaglandin synthesis, whether resulting from inhibition by
aspirin-like drugs, or increases induced by either acute stress
(5), infusion of arachidonic acid (8), or administration of a
loop diuretic (2), are likely to be reflected primarily by
alterations of that portion of renal blood flow which supplies
the medulla and will be reflected by decreased or increased blood
flow to the inner and mid cortex, as measured by the distribution
of radioactive microspheres within the cortex. This effect of
altered prostaglandin synthesis on zonal distribution of renal
blood flow arises from two factors. First, stratification of
prostaglandin synthetase intrarenally is opposite to that of
renin; the greatest prostaglandin synthetic capacity is in the
papilla and medulla, the least in the renal cortex (9). It
should be noted that the apparent difference in prostaglandin
biosynthetic capacity between the renal cortex and medulla may be
related, in part, to the presence within the cortex of an inhibitor of cyclooxygenase (10). Second, the inner cortical and
medullary circulations are continuous, as the afferent arterioles
of the inner cortex extend into the medulla, giving rise to the
vasa recta (11). Therefore, changes in prostaglandin synthesis
in the inner medulla will have secondary effects on blood flow to
the outer medulla and inner and mid cortex because of the morpho-
logical unity of these vascular structures. A possible clinical
correlation of these findings is the nephropathy of analgesic
abuse. Nanra et al have proposed that "analgesic-nephropathy" is
due to medullary ischemia secondary to reduced synthesis of one
or more vasodilator prostaglandin(s) (12), such as PGE_2 or PGI_2.
Further, elevated tissue levels of PGE_2, the presumed agent of
enhanced renomedullary blood flow, should result from inhibition
of PGE-9-ketoreductase. Furosemide and ethacrynic acid have been
shown to inhibit this enzyme and should thereby promote increased
renal blood flow to the medulla (13).
The evidence for a prostaglandin mechanism participating in
the regulation of the intrarenal distribution of blood flow was
first obtained in the isolated blood-perfused kidney of the dog

(14) - and later in the conscious rabbit (15). One or more renal prostaglandin(s), primarily PGE_2, is responsible for mediating increases in blood flow to the renal medulla in response to stimuli as diverse as surgical trauma (5), hemorrhagic hypotension (4), salt loading (16), and loop diuretic agents (17). Those interventions which increase prostaglandin production, even though they may reduce total renal blood flow, can increase blood flow to the renal medulla. A balanced mechanism seems to regulate the distribution of renal blood flow: a prostaglandin mechanism increases blood flow to the inner cortex and medulla, and one of the components of the renin-angiotensin system, angiotensin I, probably has a major intrarenal role effecting decreases in blood flow to the medulla (18). This action on the intrarenal distribution of blood flow may be unique for angiotensin I, as angiotensin II usually results in reduction in renal blood flow to all zones (18). It should be noted that high doses of angiotensin II, which can stimulate prostaglandin synthesis, may cause an increase in medullary blood flow despite a decline in total renal blood flow. As diuretic agents have the capacity to activate the renin-angiotensin system consequent to reduction of extracellular fluid volume, some of the effects on renal hemodynamics may operate through this mechanism.

In contrast to its effect on the surgically-stressed anesthetized dog, indomethacin did not affect renal blood flow in the conscious resting dog, even in doses having major toxic effects (5). This finding supports the proposal that, under physiological conditions, those mechanisms involving renal prostaglandins are quiescent, requiring a noxious stimulus to be activated. This proposal also is in agreement with the general conclusion that prostaglandins subserve a defensive function, and that their release from an organ represents synthesis on demand, as prostaglandins are not stored (1). Although this conclusion appears valid for many tissues, it fails to explain the basal efflux, albeit low, of prostaglandins from kidneys of the conscious resting dog, which is unaffected by high doses of indomethacin (5). Further, in the conscious rabbit (15) and perhaps in resting man (19), inhibition of prostaglandin synthesis has been shown to result in increased vascular resistance. In the conscious rabbit, indomethacin increased renal vascular resistance two-fold, associated with a shift of renal blood flow to the outer cortex (15). Thus, the activity of intrarenal prostaglandin mechanisms in the conscious animal under physiological conditions may vary with the species. Nasjletti et al (20) have obtained evidence that the release of prostaglandins from the kidney under resting conditions is determined, in large part, by the activity of the renal kallikrein-kinin system.

PROSTAGLANDIN BIOSYNTHETIC CAPACITY OF RENAL TISSUES

An alternative explanation for the failure of indomethacin

to affect renal blood flow in the conscious resting dog derives
from possible differences in accessibility of aspirin-like
compounds to prostaglandin synthetase, perhaps reflecting variation in metabolism or distribution of the inhibitor. Another
explanation is that the cyclooxygenase varies in its suscep-
tibility to aspirin-like drugs depending on the tissue and
species; this seems less likely (21). Thus, the question of
access of indomethacin to its site of action, as well as species
and tissue differences in the effects of indomethacin on the
prostaglandin synthesizing machinery, must be kept in mind. This
consideration leads to an important observation; viz., the
capacity to synthesize prostaglandins is distributed widely among
the cellular elements of the kidney. Cyclooxygenase is present
in at least three different tissues in the kidney. The interstitial cells of the renal medulla were the first to be shown to
have the capacity to synthesize prostaglandins (21). Also,
cyclooxygenase was shown to be localized in the cells lining the
distal nephron and collecting ducts (22); this location accords
with the known interrelationships of prostaglandins and ADH (23).
(Figure 1). For example, increased urinary concentrating ability
in response to ADH occurred after treatment with indomethacin
(24). Prostaglandins of the E series have been shown to blunt
the effects of ADH (23) and favor the excretion of free water. A
prostaglandin mechanism may contribute to the action of those
diuretic agents which increase levels of PGE_2 in the renal
medulla. The latter could be effected by an action of the
diuretic agent either on synthesis of prostaglandins, or on the
enzyme 15-hydroxyprostaglandin dehydrogenase which degrades PGE_2
or by inhibition of PGE-9-ketoreductase which transforms PGE_2 to
$PGF_{2\alpha}$. Indeed, furosemide may have effects on each of these
mechanisms; it increases prostaglandin synthesis by promoting
arachidonic acid delivery to the cyclooxygenase (25) and inhibits
both the dehydrogenase and reductase (13). The $NADP^+$-dependent
form of the dehydrogenase has been suggested to be identical to
the PGE-9-ketoreductase (26).

POSSIBLE CIRCULATING PROSTAGLANDINS

        There is little evidence that prostaglandins function as
circulating hormones. An exception to this was thought to be
PGA_2 which, when infused intravenously, was not destroyed on
passage across the pulmonary circulation (31). However, in all
probability, PGA_2 is an artifact resulting from spontaneous
breakdown of PGE_2 during extraction and purification of tissues
or plasma; recent studies based on highly sensitive and specific
mass spectrometric methods did not detect PGA_2 in the blood (32).
Recently, PGI_2 has been suggested to function as a circulating
hormone because its vasodepressor activity is undiminished by
passage across the lung (33).

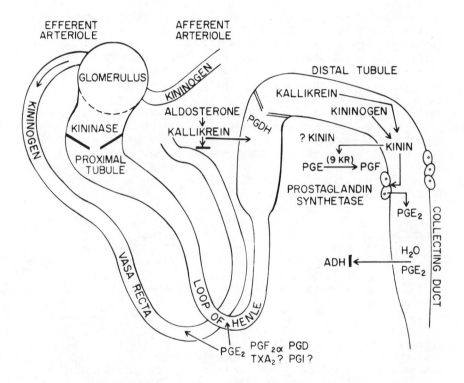

Figure 1.   Prostaglandin–kinin interaction in the nephron.

The generation of kinins in the distal nephron and collecting ducts results in the release of prostaglandins which inhibit the effect of ADH and thereby participate in the excretion of solute-free water.   Prostaglandin-15-hydroxydehydrogenase (PGHD), PGE-9-ketoreductase (9 KR).

RENAL ANATOMICAL COMPARTMENTS: PROSTAGLANDINS AND RENAL FUNCTION

Although cyclooxygenase is present in many tissues within
the kidney, the major products of arachidonic acid metabolism, be
they PGI_2, PGE_2, PGD_2, $PGF_{2\alpha}$, or TXA_2 (Figure 2), may be tissue
specific and, consequently, their effects may be primarily
restricted to one compartment, such as the vascular, tubular or
interstitial. Thus, prostacyclin, a major product of arachidonic
acid metabolism within the blood vessel wall (34), which together
with other prostaglandins may affect the activity of the renin-
angiotensin system, is possibly destroyed locally by the abundant
prostaglandin dehydrogenases of the vascular tissues (27). The
renin-angiotensin system is primarily restricted to the vascular
compartment as is prostacyclin. This is in contrast to kallikrein-kinin and PGE_2 which are mainly associated with the urinary
and interstitial compartments. Thus, the presence of prostaglandin synthetase within one or more cellular elements lining
the urinary compartment, particularly the distal nephron and
collecting ducts (22), facilitates the interaction of prostaglandins with kinins and ADH. For example, entry of kallikrein
into the distal tubules, and subsequent formation of kinins,
results in release of one or more prostaglandins by kinins from
sites of prostaglandin generation along the collecting ducts.
Inhibition of the effects of ADH can occur, then, in response to
the kinin-mediated generation of prostaglandins in the distal
nephron; this results in the excretion of solute-free water. A
recent study by Weber et al (36) indicates that the activity of a
major prostaglandin metabolizing enzyme (37), PGE-9-ketoreduc-
tase, which converts PGE_2 to $PGF_{2\alpha}$, is influenced by salt intake.
Thus, reabsorption of water is facilitated by increased activity
of this enzyme, which has the effect of lowering levels of PGE_2
intrarenally by favoring formation of $PGF_{2\alpha}$. As $PGF_{2\alpha}$, unlike
PGE_2, does not inhibit ADH, increased activity of PGE-9-keto-
reductase will facilitate reabsorption in water. The "loop
diuretic" agents have already been noted to be capable of in-
hibiting the activity of this enzyme. It should be noted that
kinins, in addition to promoting prostaglandin synthesis, are
also capable of increasing the activity of PGE-9-ketoreductase
(38), and that these effects may be crucial to the ability of
kinins to alter excretion of solute-free water as affected by the
state of sodium balance. As inhibition of prostaglandin synthesis has been shown to prevent increased free water generation
induced by bradykinin (39), a prostaglandin mechanism appears to
be necessary for this effect of the kinin (Figure 1).

PROSTAGLANDINS AND SALT EXCRETION

The concept of segregation of cyclooxygenases within several
functional compartments of the kidney and different prostaglandins arising from these compartments is useful for

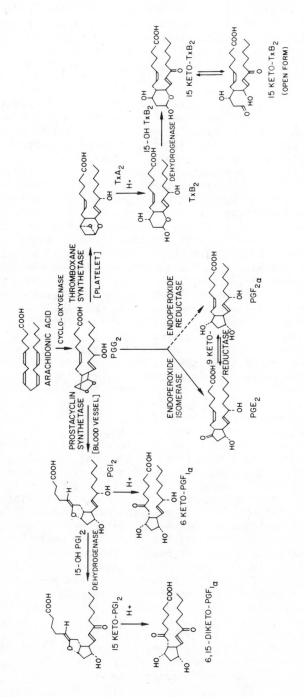

Figure 2. Metabolism of arachidonic acid by the prostaglandin synthetase complex.

Major products of vascular tissues are prostacyclin (PGI$_2$) and PGE$_2$; a major product of blood platelets is thromboxane A$_2$ (TxA$_2$)

interpreting the variable effects of one or more prostaglandin
mechanisms on salt excretion. The natriuretic effect of either
the principal renal prostaglandin, PGE_2, or its precursor,
arachidonic acid, cannot be dissociated easily from its effects
on the renal circulation. In the only in vivo study which
examined the effect of PGE_2 on tubular function uncomplicated by
vascular effects, Kauker, using micro-injection techniques,
demonstrated that intraluminal injection of PGE_2 in rats resulted
in inhibition of sodium reabsorption (40). Further, Stokes and
Kokko demonstrated an inhibitory effect of PGE_2 on sodium transport in isolated perfused renal collecting tubules of rabbits
pretreated with mineralocorticoids (41). In conscious rats,
Nasjletti et al (20) demonstrated that mineralocorticoid treatment not only increased kallikrein excretion, but also enhanced
excretion of PGE_2 by two- to three-fold. Augmented excretion of
kallikrein and PGE_2 in these rats was associated with escape from
the salt and water retaining effects of mineralocorticoids. In
the rat, inhibition of prostaglandin synthesis also results in
increased concentration of sodium chloride in the renal medulla
(42). The latter suggests that exaggerated tubular reabsorption
of sodium in the ascending limb of the loop of Henle results from
eliminating a prostaglandin mechanism which promotes salt excretion. On the other hand, in the conscious dog undergoing a
water-induced diuresis, both indomethacin and meclofenamate have
been reported to increase sodium excretion (43). A possible
prostaglandin mechanism which prevents demonstration of the
direct natriuretic action of bradykinin was described by McGiff
et al in the blood-perfused isolated canine kidney (39). Thus, a
natriuretic action of bradykinin was not shown until prostaglandin synthesis was inhibited by indomethacin. These seemingly
discrepant studies may be reconciled if it is recognized that the
experimental conditions determine not only the level of prostaglandin activity, but also the major species of prostaglandins
produced within the urinary compartment. As these vary, the
effects of indomethacin, which also alters prostaglandin metabolizing enzymes (13), will depend on the level and profile of
prostaglandins produced under a given set of conditions. This,
in turn, is related to the state of salt and water balance, the
degree of stress occasioned by anesthesia and surgery, the
activity of other hormonal systems, the "intrinsic" activity of
the cyclooxygenase as determined by natural inhibitors and
activators, and, finally, the species being studied. These
general considerations force the conclusion that the products of
cyclooxygenases in the various compartments within the kidney may
vary with experimental conditions, as well as in health and in
disease. For example, thromboxane, a powerful vasoconstrictor; is
not normally synthesized by the kidney. However, when renal
function is disturbed, as by acute ureteral ligation, thromboxane
synthesis may occur (44). Its production may contribute to the
late increase in renal vascular resistance in response to

ureteral obstruction (45).

Changes in extracellular potassium concentration can also affect renal prostaglandin synthesis (46). As urinary kallikrein concentrations have been positively correlated with excretion of potassium, but not sodium (47), the possibility of a potassium-dependent interaction of prostaglandins with kallikrein-kinins should be considered. Thus, induction of potassium deficiency has been shown to result in enhanced renal prostaglandin synthesis (48). Hyposthenuria associated with potassium deficiency, then, may be related to inhibition of the effects of ADH (23) consequent to increased production of PGE_2 or a related prostaglandin.

SUMMARY

Those diuretic agents such as furosemide which have as their primary sites of action the ascending limb of the loop of Henle and the cortical collecting ducts, where they have a primary effect on chloride transport (49), can be shown to have major effects not only on the renin-angiotensin system (6), but also on the kallikrein-kinin (50) and prostaglandin systems (13). There is evidence suggesting that their diuretic action may be related partially to an effect on the vasodilator-diuretic system of the kidney, the kallikrein-kinin-prostaglandin system. Thus, aspirin-like compounds have been shown to blunt the diuretic action of furosemide (51), although this effect of antiinflammatory acids is complicated by their inhibition of the organic acid secretory system. Integrity of the latter may be required for access of these diuretic agents to their active sites. Further, furosemide and ethacrynic acid have been shown to inhibit two of the major prostaglandin catabolizing enzymes, prostaglandin-15-hydroxydehydrogenase and PGE-9-ketoreductase (13). Their effects on these enzymes may result in increased levels of PGE_2 and PGI_2 which may then contribute to vasodilator-diuretic mechanisms. The design of agents which have major effects on prostaglandin metabolism is well underway and has already resulted in novel diuretic agents (52).

Acknowledgments - We thank Mrs. Cathy Reynolds and Mrs. Sue Hatton for assistance in typing the manuscript. This study was supported by USPHS Grants HL-18845 and HL-22075 and American Heart Association Grant 77-987.

Literature Cited

1. Änggard, E., Bohman, S. O., Griffin, J. E., III, Larsson, C., and Maunsbach, A. B., Acta Physiol. Scand. (1972), 84, 231-246.
2. Olsen, U. B., Acta Pharmacol. Toxicol. (1977), 41, 1-31.
3. McGiff, J. C., Crowshaw, K., Terragno, N. A., and Lonigro, A., Nature (1970), 227, 1255-1257.
4. Vatner, S. F., J. Clin. Invest. (1974), 54, 225-235.
5. Terragno, N. A., Terragno, D. A. and McGiff, J. C. Circ. Res. (1977), 40, 590-595.

6. Bailie, M.D., Davis, L. E. and Loutzenhiser, R., Am. J. Physiol (1973), 224, 425-430.

7. Itskovitz, H. D., Terragno, N. A. and McGiff, J. C., Circ. Res. (1974), 34, 770-776.

8. Chang, L. C. T., Splawinski, J. A., Oates, J. A. and Nies, A. S., Circ. Res. (1975), 36, 204-207.

9. Larsson, C. and Änggard, E., Eur. J. Pharmacol. (1974), 21, 30-36.

10. Terragno, N. A., McGiff, J. C. and Terragno, A., Clin. Res. (1978), 26, 545A (abstract).

11. Fourman, J. and Moffat, D. B., "Blood Vessels of the Kidney", p. 58, Oxford, Blackwell Scientific Publications, Oxford, England, 1971.

12. Nanra, R. S., Chirawong, P. and Kincaid-Smith, P., Aust. N. Z. Med. (1973), 3, 580-586.

13. Stone, K. J. and Hart, M., Prostaglandins (1976), 12, 197-207.

14. Itskovitz, H. D., Stemper, J., Pacholczyk, D. and McGiff, J. C., Clin. Sci. (1973), 45, 321s-324s.

15. Beilin, L. J. and Bhattacharya, J., J. Physiol. (1977), 269, 395-405.

16. Papanicolaou, N., Safar, M., Hornych, A., Fontaliran, F., Weiss, Y., Bariety, J. and Milliez, P., Clin. Sci. Molec. Med. (1975), 49, 459-463.

17. Olsen, U. B. and Ahnfelt-Ronne, I. Acta Physiol. Scand. (1976), 97, 251-257.

18. Itskovitz, H. and McGiff, J. C., Circ. Res. (1974), 34-35, (Suppl I), 65-73.

19. Wennmalm, A., IRCS (1974), 2, 1099.

20. Nasjletti, A., McGiff, J. C. and Colina-Chourio, J., Circ. Res., in press.

21. Pong, S. S. and Levine, L., J. Pharmacol. Exp. Ther. (1976), 196-197, 226-230.

22. Smith, W. L. and Wilkin, G. P., Prostaglandins (1977), 13, 873-892.

23. Grantham, J. J. and Orloff, J., J. Clin. Invest. (1968), 47, 1154-1161.

24. Berl, P., Raz, A., Wald, H., Horowitz, J. and Czaczkes, W., Am. J. Physiol. (1977), 232, F529-F537.

25. Weber, P. C., Scherer, B. and Larsson, C., Eur. J. Pharmacol. (1977), 41, 329-332.

26. Hassid, A. and Levine, L., Prostaglandins (1977), 13, 503-516.

27. Wong, P. Y-K., Sun, F. F. and McGiff, J. C., J. Biol. Chem. (1978), in press.

28. Larsson, C., Weber, P. and Änggard, E., Eur. J. Pharmacol. (1974), 28, 391-394.

29. Gerber, J. G., Branch, R. A., Nies, A. S., Gerkens, J. F., Shand, D. G., Hollifield, J. and Oates, J. A., Prostaglandins (1978), 15, 81-88.

30. Terragno, D. A., Crowshaw, K., Terragno, N. A. and McGiff, J. C., Circ. Res. (1975), 36-37, (Suppl I), 76-80.

31. McGiff, J. C., Terragno, N. A., Strand, J. C., Lee, J. B., Lonigro, A. J. and Ng, K. K. F., Nature (1969), 223, 742-745.

32. Frolich, J. C., Sweetman, B. J., Carr, K., Hollifield, J. W. and Oates, J. A., Prostaglandins (1975), 10, 185-195.

33. Armstrong, J. M., Lattimer, N., Moncada, S. and Vane, J. R., Br. J. Pharmac. (1978), 62, 125-130.

34. Moncada, S., Gryglewski, R. J., Bunting, S. and Vane, J. R., Prostaglandins (1976), 12, 715-737.

35. Carretero, O. A. and Scicli, A. G., Fed. Proc. (1976), 35, 194-198.

36. Weber, P. C., Larsson, C. and Scherer, B., Nature (1977), 266, 65-66.

37. Leslie, C. A. and Levine, L., Biochem. Biophys. Res. Commun. (1973), 52, 717-724.

38. Wong, P. Y-K, Terragno, D. A., Terragno, N. A. and McGiff, J. C., Prostaglandins (1977), 13, 1113-1125.

39. McGiff, J. C., Itskovitz, H. D. and Terragno, N. A., Clin. Sci. Molec. Med. (1975), 49, 125-131.

40. Kauker, M. L., Proc. Soc. Exp. Biol. Med. (1977), 154, 272-277.

41. Stokes, J. B. and Kokko, J. P., J. Clin. Invest. (1977), 59, 1099-1104.

42. Ganguli, M., Tobian, L., Azar, S. and O'Donnell, M., Circ. Res. (1977), 40, (Suppl I), 135-139.

43. Kirschenbaum, M. A. and Stein, J. H., J. Clin. Invest. (1976), 57, 517-521.

44. Morrison, A., Nishikawa, K. and Needleman, P., Nature (1977), 267, 259-260.

45. Yarger, W. E. and Griffith, L. D., Am. J. Physiol. (1974), 227, 816-826.

46. Zusman, R. M. and Keiser, H. R., J. Clin. Invest. (1977), 60, 215-223.

47. Zinner, S. H., Margolius, H. S., Rosner, B., Keiser, H. R. and Kass, E. H., Am. J. Epidem. (1976), 104, 124-132.

48. Galvez, O. G., Bay, W. H., Roberts, B. W. and Ferris, R. F., Circ. Res. (1977), 40, (Suppl 9), 11-16.

49. Rocha, A. S. and Kokko, J. P., J. Clin. Invest. (1973), 52, 612-623.

50. Croxatto, H. R., Roblero, J. S., Garcia, R. L., Corthorn, J. H. and San Martin, M., Acta Physiol. Latino Am. (1973), 22-23, 556-558.

51. Lee, J. B., Proc. 6th Int. Congr. Nephrol. (1975), 1, 348-354.

52. Cragoe, E. J., Jr., Schultz, E. M., Schneeberg, J. D., Stokker, G. E., Woltersdorf, O. W., Jr., Fanelli, G. M., Jr., and Watson, L. S., J. Med. Chem. (1975), 18, 225-228.

RECEIVED August 21, 1978.

2

Structure–Activity Relationships of Aminobenzoic Acid Diuretics and Related Compounds (*1*)

O. B. TVAERMOSE NIELSEN and P. W. FEIT

Leo Pharmaceutical Products, 2750 Ballerup, Denmark

In a series of papers (2-10) during the nineteen-seventies, we presented some of our results based on a more or less systematic structural alteration of the sulfamoylbenzoic acid diuretics in order to elucidate the structural requirements for high-ceiling diuretic activity.

When we started this work, for reasons previously discussed (3), the only existing high-ceiling sulfonamide diuretics were the N-substituted 4-chloro-5-sulfamoylanthranilic acids represented by furosemide (Formula 1). Although the diuretic characteristics of furosemide were quite different from those of the thiazides or the thiazide-type diuretics, thereby reflecting a different site of action in the nephron, it still shared structural features with the latter compounds. Thus, furosemide fit the structural requirements for diuretic activity of the benzenesulfonamides and related bicyclic compounds originally proposed by Sprague (11). He predicted that an unsubstituted sulfamoyl group, an activating group represented mainly by chloro and trifluoromethyl and an electronegative substituent (which might be part of a condensed ring system) should be present in the molecule and have the mutual positions reflected in furosemide.

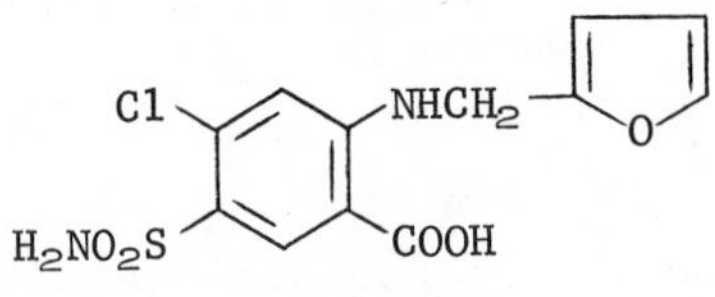

1

Our first approach was to move the substituted amino function (which is not part of Sprague's predictions) to the 3-position, with almost complete retention of diuretic activity (2). More surprisingly, replacement of the chlorine atom by various other groups in both the 2-substituted (4, 5) and the 3-substituted

0-8412-0464-0/78/47-083-**012**$05.00/0
© American Chemical Society

(3, 6, 7, 8) sulfamoylbenzoic acid diuretics, was found to enhance the diuretic potency. The most potent compounds (Formula 2) were those in which an unsubstituted or substituted phenyl group was linked to the 4-position by a group X, which represents NH, O, S, SO, SO_2, CH_2 or CO. These 4-substituents are not merely new "activating groups" in the sense that Sprague described, since replacement of chloro by phenoxy or phenylthio in some selected thiazides and thiazide-type diuretics led to compounds which were not diuretic (12). The predictions of Sprague, although still of value as far as the thiazide-type diuretics were concerned, were found not to account fully for the structural requirements of the high-ceiling diuretics.

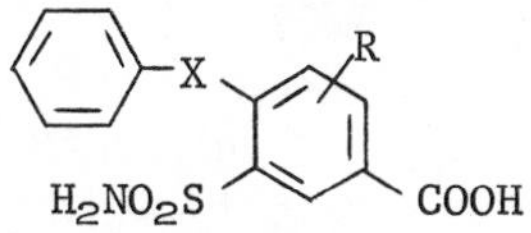

X = NH, O, S, SO, SO_2, CH_2, CO

R = NHR^1, OR^1, SR^1, CH_2R^1 in which R^1 preferably is n-butyl, benzyl, furyl-methyl or thienylmethyl

2

When placed in the 3-position, many variations of the sub-stituent R in formula 2 contribute to high potency. However, when located in the 2-position, the only active compounds are those where R is restricted to a substituted amino function, preferably the 2-furylmethylamino group.

Bumetanide (Formula 3) was selected for further investigation and shown (13) to be 40 to 60 times more potent than furosemide; this was a level of potency exhibited in the dog assay by many compounds of formula 2. Its utility in clinical practice has since been established (14).

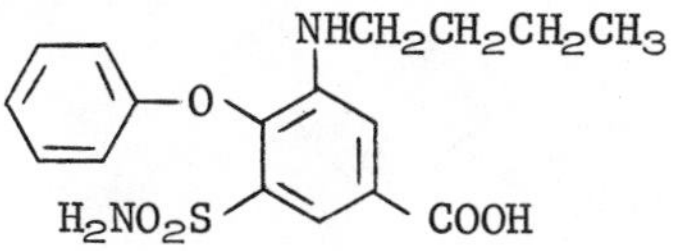

3

The compounds of formula 2, in which X represents carbonyl and R a substituted amino function, are not isolable due to a pH-dependent equilibrium in aqueous solution. At physiological pH, the equilibrium favors the cyclodehydration products, i.e., the benzisothiazole dioxides of formula 4. It has been suggested (5, 6), however, that the potent diuretic activity (one fourth to one tenth of that of bumetanide) observed after administration of these benzisothiazoles to dogs involves the interaction of the corresponding 4-benzoylsulfamoylbenzoic acids (Formula 5) with

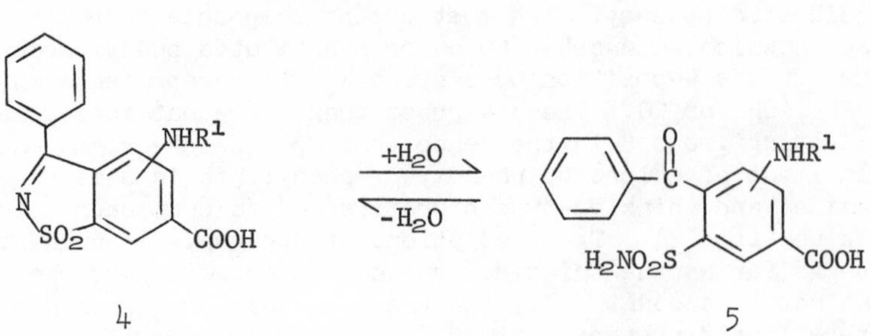

the receptor which is possible because of the dynamic equilibration in plasma. Thus, the potency of the benzisothiazole
dioxides (Formula 4) appears to be due to this remarkable property. For the corresponding 3-alkoxy- or 3-alkylthio-4-benzoyl-
5-sulfamoylbenzoic acids, the equilibrium is totally to the side
of the benzoyl compound (8); this might explain why compound 6
(Table I) is one of the most potent, high-ceiling diuretics that
we synthesized. Since this compound shows significant diuretic
activity in the dog assay after an oral dose of only 1 μg/kg, it
is 5 to 10 times more potent than bumetanide (8).

TABLE I

Urinary Excretion in a 3 hr. Period following I.V. Administration
of Compound 6 to Dogs, Expressed for Vol. in ml/kg and for
Electrolytes in mEq/kg.

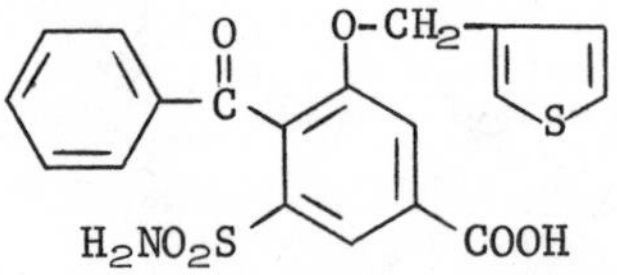

Treatment mg/kg	Vol.	Na^+	K^+	Cl^-
control	1	0.10	0.16	0.08
0.001	4	0.7	0.28	0.7
0.01	23	2.5	0.53	3.5
0.1	38	4.4	0.97	4.9

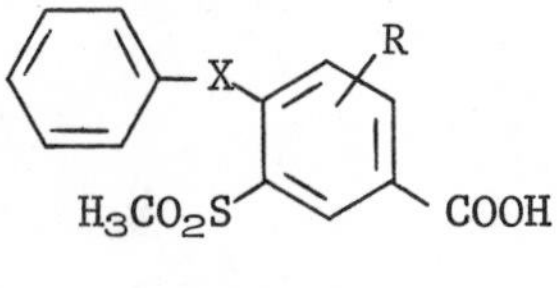

X = NH, O, S, CO

R = NHR^1, OR^1, SR^1 in which R^1
preferably is n-butyl,
benzyl or furylmethyl

7

   Another discovery was that active diuretics of the type
represented by formula 7 could be obtained when the sulfamoyl
group was replaced by the sterically similar mesyl group (9).
Various 3-substituents contribute to the comparatively high
potency of these compounds; whereas, virtually the only 2-sub-
stituent allowed is the 2-furylmethylamino group. These observations encouraged the investigation of the influence of other
substituents in the 5-position. A suitably substituted amino
function, preferably a formamido group in place of the sulfamoyl
group (Formula 8), led to active diuretics (10).

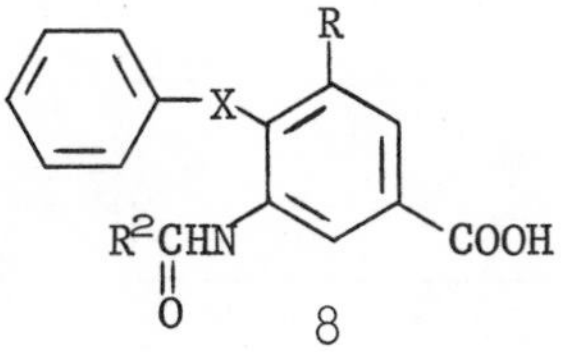

X = O, S, CH$_2$, CO

R = NHR^1, OR^1, SR^1, CH$_2$R^1 in
which R^1 preferably is
n-butyl, benzyl, furyl-
methyl or thienylmethyl.

R^2 = H, lower alkyl, NH$_2$,
NH-lower alkyl, lower
alkoxy

8

Table II shows the data obtained with one of the most potent
compounds with this particular structural alteration. Compound 9
was found to be approximately one tenth as potent as bumetanide.
Disappointingly, the electrolyte excretion pattern was still
similar to that of bumetanide. The corresponding 2,4-
disubstituted-5-acylaminobenzoic acids were, however, inactive.

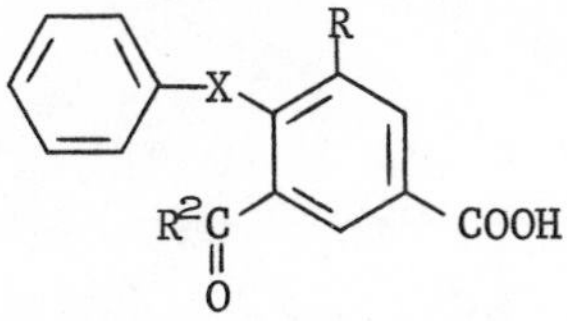

X = NH, O, S, CO
R = NHR^1, OR^1, SR^1 in which R^1
preferably is n-butyl or
benzyl

R^2 = OH, NH$_2$, NH-lower alkyl

10

TABLE II

Urinary Excretion (Average of 3 Values) in a 3 hr. Period
following I.V. Administration of Compound 9 to Dogs, Expressed
for Vol. in ml/kg and for Electrolytes in mEq/kg.

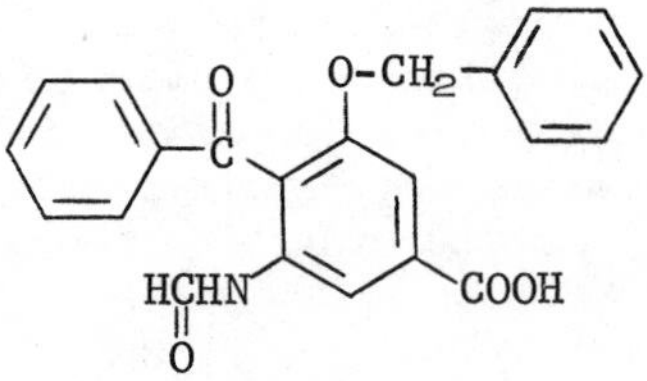

9

Treatment mg/kg	Vol.	Na^+	K^+	Cl^-
control	1	0.10	0.16	0.08
0.1	9	1.0	0.24	1.3
0.25	18	2.1	0.41	2.6
1.0	22	2.5	0.49	3.1
5.0	32	3.7	0.83	4.5

   In addition, isophthalic acid derivatives of formula 10 were
prepared (15). Some of them exerted moderate diuretic activity;
however, again, the characteristic electrolyte excretion profile
of bumetanide was observed.
   The above brief survey of previously reported results of
structural modifications in benzoic acid diuretics reveals that
our efforts had been directed toward compounds in which the
carboxylic acid function remained intact. If such a function is
present in biologically active molecules, its acidic character
usually has, for known reasons, an effect on activity and/or
potency. Therefore, it was considered to be of interest to
investigate whether a carboxyl function is a prerequisite for
high-ceiling diuretic activity. Consequently, derivatives in
which this group was replaced by other functions were synthesized.
   3,4-Disubstituted-5-sulfamoylbenzenesulfinic acids and sulfonic acids of formula 11 (Table III) were prepared from the
corresponding carboxylic acids. Conversion of their azides by
means of a Curtius degradation furnished the corresponding ani-
lines. The latter derivatives were converted to the sulfonyl
chlorides via diazotization and the Meerwein-reaction. These were
subsequently hydrolyzed to sulfonic acids or reduced to sulfinic
acids. It can be seen from Table III that these rather strong
acids possess potent diuretic activity. Their diuretic profile is
quite similar to that of bumetanide; however, they have a shorter
duration of action. The corresponding 2,4,5-trisubstituted acids
were not investigated since, 15 years previously, the sulfinic
acid analogue of furosemide had been found by us to be devoid of
activity at a dose of 10 mg/kg in the dog assay. In contrast,
3-butylamino-4-chloro-5-sulfamoylbenzenesulfinic acid was found to
be diuretic at a dose of 1 mg/kg.
   A series of 3,4-disubstituted-5-sulfamoylbenzylamines was
synthesized (16). In the dog assay, many of these compounds
exhibited high-ceiling diuretic activity in the range of potency
from that of furosemide to that of bumetanide. Therefore, an
extended series of benzylamines of formula 12 (see Table IV)
having the 3-, 4-, and 5-substituents of bumetanide was prepared
in order to elucidate the influence of the N-substituent(s) in the
benzylamine moiety on diuretic activity. Selected members of this
series are tabulated in Table IV. It appears that many R^2 and R^3
substituents, such as hydrogen, lower straight chain alkyl, allyl,
benzyl, furylmethyl, pyridylmethyl and unsubstituted as well as
suitably substituted phenyl, contribute to high potency. Disubstitution, as exemplified by N,N-dimethyl, N,N-diethyl and some
N-alkyl, N-hydroxyethyl derivatives, also is an allowed structural
modification. In contrast, incorporation of a nitrogen atom in a
ring system to provide derivatives of piperidine, morpholine and
N'-substituted piperazine results in compounds which are inactive
at the doses tested. Likewise, substitution with branched alkyl,
acyl, carbamoyl or N-substituted carbamoyl groups generally
decreases or abolishes diuretic activity.

TABLE III

Urinary Excretion in a 6 hr. Period following I.V. Administration
to Dogs of 1 mg/kg Expressed for Vol. in ml/kg and for
Electrolytes in mEq/kg.

11

X	R	n	Vol.	Na^+	K^+	Cl^-
	Control (extreme values from 108 exp.)		0.3-4.2	0.05 - 0.45	0.06 - 0.30	0.06 - 0.28
O	NHC_4H_9	2	37	4.1	1.02	5.3
O	$NHCH_2C_6H_5$	2	48	4.7	1.05	4.5
O	SC_4H_9	2	29	4.0	1.15	1.7
CH_2	OC_4H_9	2	34	3.0	1.31	5.2
O	NHC_4H_9	3	22	2.6	0.62	3.1
O	$NHCH_2C_6H_5$	3	48	4.3	0.91	6.6
O	N⬠	3	35	3.3	0.91	4.1

Various 3- and 4-substituents, found in the series of benzoic acids of formula 2 to contribute to high-ceiling potency, were incorporated in a series of compounds in which the variation of the benzylamine moiety was restricted to selected N-substituents. Since the influence of these N-substituents did not deviate from that observed in the series of bumetanide analogues, only the results obtained with compounds of formula 13 having the benzyl-amino nitrogen atom substituted by phenyl are given in Table V. As previously observed with the benzoic acid diuretics of formula 2, groups such as R^1O, R^1S or R^1NH (where R^1 is n-butyl, benzyl, furylmethyl or thienylmethyl) placed in the 3-position enhanced the diuretic activity. Likewise, phenyl attached to the 4-position through the well-known links, NH, O, S or CH_2, also was found to contribute to the potent high-ceiling diuretic activity of the benzylamine series.

A number of 2,4-disubstituted-5-sulfamoylbenzylamines having as the 2-substituent the outstanding 2-furylmethylamino group of furosemide and related anthranilic acids were found to be inactive. This lack of activity might well be due to an inadmissible structural modification. However, after administration of selected 3-substituted benzylamines to dogs, the presence of the corresponding benzoic acids in the urine has been demonstrated qualitatively. Consequently, the question arises as to whether the diuretic response following treatment with 3-substituted benzylamines should be explained solely on the basis of metabolic transformation to the corresponding benzoic acid diuretics of formula 2. The marked difference in diuretic activity between the 2-substituted and the 3-substituted benzylamines could be due only to the repressed metabolism of the 2-derivatives due to the steric effect of the ortho-substituent. On the other hand, the above mentioned effects on diuretic activity may be accounted for by the similar differences between the 2- and the 3-substituted derivatives in the 5-acylaminobenzoic series and between the 2- and 3-substituted-4-chloro-5-sulfamoylbenzenesulfinic acid series. Furthermore, the inconsistency between the observed diuretic activities and the rate at which the subject benzylamines (Table IV) would be expected to be metabolized, might support the view that the 3-substituted benzylamines possess intrinsic diuretic activity.

The only conclusions we dare to draw from the results of our research during more than a decade in the exciting field of diuretics are that numerous structural alterations of disubstituted sulfamoylbenzoic acid diuretics led to compounds with highly potent high-ceiling diuretic activity, and that the 3,4-disubstituted members of this series are less sensitive to such alterations than are the 2,4-disubstituted members. Further exploration in this area might still, in our opinion, uncover benzene ring substituents or substitution patterns leading to compounds with high-ceiling diuretic activity.

Acknowledgment - The authors are greatly indebted to the

TABLE IV

Urinary Excretion (Mean of 2 Values) in a 6 hr. Period following
I.V. (when marked with an asterisk p.o.) Administration to Dogs
of 1 mg/kg, Expressed for Vol. in ml/kg and for Electrolytes
in mEq/kg.

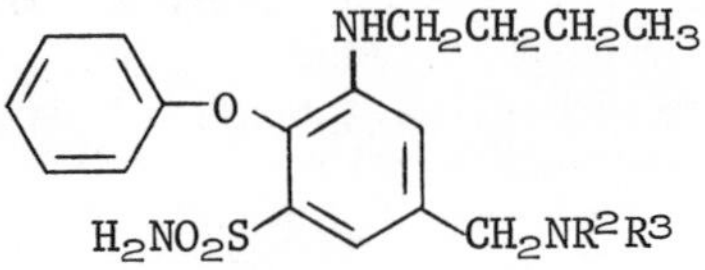

$$NHCH_2CH_2CH_2CH_3$$

benzene ring with O-phenyl, H_2NO_2S, and $CH_2NR^2R^3$ substituents

12

R^2	R^3	Vol.	Na^+	K^+	Cl^-
Control (extreme values from 108 exp.)		0.3 – 4.2	0.05 – 0.45	0.06 – 0.30	0.06 – 0.28
H	H	23	4.5	0.81	2.6
methyl	H	19	1.5	0.35	2.4
ethyl	H	17	2.0	0.48	2.4
n-propyl	H	*17	1.9	0.67	2.6
isopropyl	H	12	0.8	0.32	0.7
allyl	H	29	3.5	1.3	3.7
$CH_2C(CH_3)=CH_2$	H	20	1.4	0.35	2.1
n-butyl	H	8	1.4	0.42	1.6
isobutyl	H	3	0.4	0.30	0.2
sec-butyl	H	5	0.4	0.09	0.4
tert-butyl	H	*7	1.1	0.27	1.2
isopentyl	H	3	0.3	0.13	0.2
n-hexyl	H	9	1.1	0.75	0.6
CH_2CH_2OH	H	3	0.3	0.18	0.3
$CH_2CHOHCH_3$	H	9	1.0	0.39	1.1
$CH_2CH_2NEt_2$	H	1	0.1	0.05	0.1
methyl	methyl	21	2.1	0.48	2.6
ethyl	ethyl	10	1.0	0.37	1.2
n-propyl	n-propyl	*4	0.5	0.21	0.6
methyl	CH_2CH_2OH	3	0.5	0.18	0.4
ethyl	CH_2CH_2OH	13	1.3	0.32	1.9
isopropyl	CH_2CH_2OH	15	1.5	0.47	2.0
$CH_2C_6H_5$	H	33	3.1	1.02	4.5
$CH_2C_6H_4$-4-Me	H	3	0.4	0.16	0.5
$CH_2C_6H_4$-3-Cl	H	*11	1.1	0.24	1.4

Table IV (Continued)

R_2	R_3	Vol.	Na^+	K^+	Cl^-
$CH_2C_6H_4$-3-OH	H	7	0.8	0.22	0.6
$CH_2C_6H_4$-4-OMe	H	11	0.8	0.25	1.3
$CH_2C_6H_5$	methyl	6	0.8	0.40	1.0
CH_2-(furanyl)	H	19	2.8	0.86	1.9
CH_2-(tetrahydrofuranyl)	H	16	1.0	0.31	1.1
CH_2-(pyridyl, N-2)	H	25	2.6	0.67	2.9
CH_2-(pyridyl, N-3)	H	16	1.7	0.46	2.1
CH_2-(pyridyl, N-4)	H	2	0.3	0.11	0.2
CH_2-(furanyl)	methyl	7	0.6	0.38	0.7
CH_2-(tetrahydrofuranyl)	methyl	7	0.9	0.26	0.9
C_6H_5	H	33	4.5	1.15	5.4
C_6H_4-2-Me	H	21	2.0	0.45	3.7
C_6H_4-4-Me	H	9	0.8	0.23	0.7
C_6H_4-2-CF_3	H	5	0.2	0.09	0.2
C_6H_4-3-F	H	4	0.5	0.15	0.3
C_6H_4-3-Cl	H	2	0.2	0.11	0.2
C_6H_4-4-Br	H	13	1.1	0.37	1.9
C_6H_4-2-OH	H	6	0.5	0.14	0.5
C_6H_4-4-OH	H	14	1.2	0.39	1.5
C_6H_4-2-OCH_3	H	2	0.2	0.32	0.2
C_6H_4-3-OC_2H_5	H	3	0.2	0.18	0.2
N-(piperidino)		*4	0.2	0.12	0.2
N-(morpholino)		5	0.7	0.48	1.1
NR^2R^3 = N-(4-methylpiperazino) N-CH_3		3	0.2	0.31	0.2
N-(4-hydroxyethylpiperazino) N-CH_2CH_2OH		3	0.4	0.22	0.3
$COCH_3$	H	2	0.3	0.14	0.1
$CONH_2$	H	1	0.1	0.10	0.1
$CONHCH_3$	H	8	0.7	0.59	0.7
$CONHC_3H_7$	H	8	1.0	0.39	1.0

TABLE V

Urinary Excretion (Mean of 2 Values) in a 6 hr. Period
following I.V. Administration to Dogs of 1 mg/kg,
Expressed for Vol. in ml/kg and for Electrolytes
in mEq/kg.

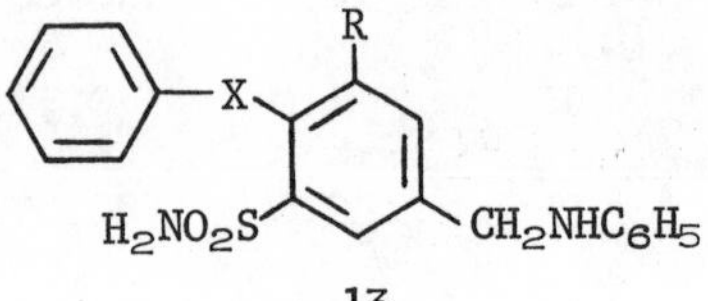

13

X	R	Vol.	Na^+	K^+	Cl^-
Control (extreme values from 108 exp.)		0.3 – 4.2	0.05 – 0.45	0.06 – 0.30	0.06 – 0.28
O	$NHCH_2CH=CH_2$	3	0.5	0.31	0.3
O	$NHCH_2C\equiv CH$	5	0.5	0.15	0.4
O	$NHCH_2CH=CHCH_3$	7	0.9	0.43	0.9
O	$NHCH_2CH_2CH_2CH_3$	33	4.5	1.15	5.4
O	$NH(CH_2)_4CH_3$	4	0.5	0.20	0.4
O	$NHCH_2C_6H_5$	25	3.0	1.3	3.8
O	$NHCH_2$ 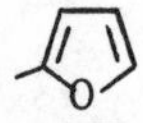 (furyl)	12	1.4	0.52	0.9
O	$NHCH_2$ 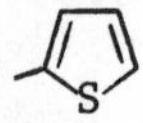 (thienyl)	28	3.2	0.83	2.2
S	$NHCH_2C_6H_5$	20	2.4	0.68	2.4
NH	$NHCH_2C_6H_5$	11	1.3	0.46	1.0
CH_2	$NHCH_2CH_2CH_2CH_3$	7	1.0	0.33	0.7
CH_2	$NHCH_2C_6H_5$	19	2.8	0.64	2.0
CH_2	$OCH_2CH_2CH_2CH_3$	14	1.9	0.61	1.4
CH_2	$OCH_2C_6H_5$	16	2.1	0.40	2.0

staff of the Department of Pharmacology and to the Huntingdon
Research Centre, Huntingdon, England, for the diuretic screening.

Literature Cited

1. Presented in part at the 174th National Meeting of the
American Chemical Society, Division of Medicinal Chemistry,
Chicago, Illinois, August–September, 1977.
2. Feit, P. W., Bruun, H. and Nielsen, C. K., J. Med. Chem.
(1970), 13, 1071.
3. Feit, P. W., J. Med. Chem. (1971), 14, 432.
4. Feit, P. W. and Nielsen, O. B. T., J. Med. Chem. (1972),
15, 79.
5. Feit, P. W., Nielsen, O. B. T. and Rastrup-Andersen, N.,
J. Med. Chem. (1973), 16, 127.
6. Nielsen, O. B. T., Nielsen, C. K. and Feit, P. W., J.
Med. Chem. (1973), 16, 1170.
7. Feit, P. W., Nielsen, O. B. T. and Bruun, H., J. Med.
Chem. (1974), 17, 572.
8. Nielsen, O. B. T., Bruun, H., Bretting, C. and Feit, P.
W., J. Med. Chem. (1975), 18, 41.
9. Feit, P. W. and Nielsen, O. B. T., J. Med. Chem. (1976),
19, 402.
10. Feit, P. W. and Nielsen, O. B. T., J. Med. Chem. (1977),
20, 1687.
11. Sprague, J. M. in "Topics in Medicinal Chemistry," Vol.
II, pp. 22–24, Rabinowitz, J. L. and Myerson, R. M., Ed.,
Wiley, New York, N. Y., 1968.
12. Feit, P. W., Nielsen, O. B. T. and Bruun, H., J. Med.
Chem. (1972), 15, 437.
13. Østergaard, E. H., Magnussen, M. P., Nielsen, C. K.,
Eilertsen, E. and Frey, H.-H., Arzneim. Forsch. (1972), 22,
66.
14. Postgrad. Med. J. (1975), 51, Suppl. 6, "Bumetanide,"
Hoffbrand, B. I. and Jones, G., Ed.
15. Feit, P. W. and Bruun, H., U.S. Patent 3,864,385 (1973).
16. Feit, P. W., Nielsen, O. B. T., Bretting, C. and Bruun,
H., U.S. Patent 4,082,851 (1978).

RECEIVED August 21, 1978.

3

4-(3-Sulfamoylphenyl)thiazolidin-4-ols

A Novel Class of Sulfonamide Compounds with Salidiuretic Activity

H.-J. LANG, B. KNABE, R. MUSCHAWECK, M. HROPOT, and E. LINDNER

Hoechst Aktiengesellschaft, Postfach 80 03 20, D-6230 Frankfurt/M. 80, West Germany

Along with other developments, the history of pharmaceutical research in our laboratories shows a close connection with the history of diuretics. A few years after the discovery in 1919 that antibiotic mercury compounds display diuretic effects (1, 2), investigators at Hoechst developed Salyrgan as the reference compound of the "Mercurials" (3). About 30 years ago, these organometallic drugs were displaced by sulfonamide derivatives which produced long acting diuresis (4, 5, 6). In 1959, researchers at Hoechst discovered the first potent short acting high-ceiling diuretic with a benzenesulfonamide structure, furosemide (7). Another interesting development in the field of high-ceiling diuretics was the synthesis of the acylphenoxyacetic acid derivative, ethacrynic acid (8). Another significant contribution to the high-ceiling diuretics which emanated from research in our laboratories was the development of piretanide (Hoe 118) during the last few years (9).

The present report will show the importance we attach to the long acting salidiuretics. When we first began our research into long acting diuretics, only the sulfonamide derivatives were known. At that time all commercial diuretics with a thiadiazide-like salidiuretic action could be derived from two general formulas, i.e., either from 3-sulfamoylsulfonamides (Structure 1) or from 3-sulfamoylbenzamides (Structure 2). Chlorthalidone (Compound 3) was an exception to this generalization (Scheme I).

Scheme I

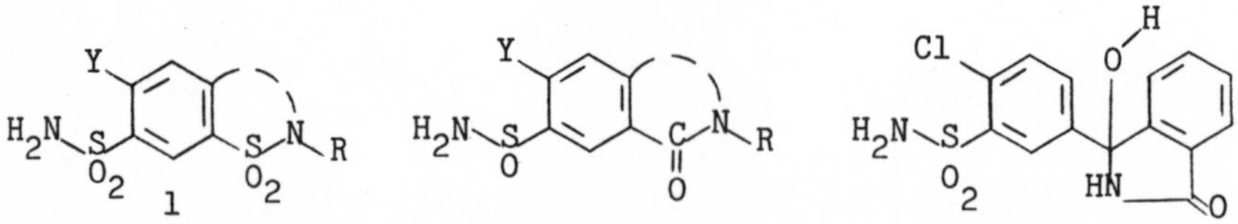

3-Sulfamoyl-sulfonamides 1

3-Sulfamoylbenzamides 2

Chlorthalidone 3

0-8412-0464-0/78/47-083-**024**$05.00/0
© American Chemical Society

As very little was known about the structure-activity relationships of chlorthalidone (10), we were interested in elucidating
the structural features which are important for the salidiuretic
activity. That is, what is the significance of the fused aryl
moiety, the carbamoyl moiety, the five membered ring, and the
N-C-OH moiety with respect to the salidiuretic activity?

Compounds 4a and 4b (Scheme II) show chlorthalidone and its
open chain tautomeric form (10).

Scheme II

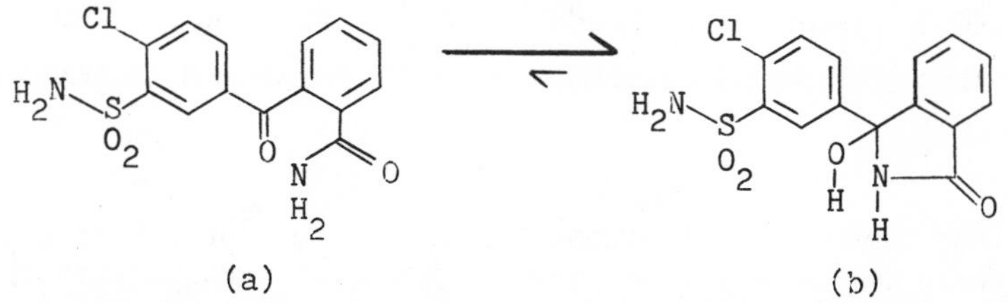

(a)   (b)

To answer our first question as to the importance of the fused
aryl moiety, we decided to prepare dearyl compounds (Scheme III)
from α-haloacetophenones (Structure 5) and bifunctional molecules
(Structure 6), where A represents the more nucleophilic portion of
this molecule. The B-H portion of Structure 7b is then free to
cyclize with the ketone carbonyl group giving ring form (Structure
7a) which would exist in tautomeric equilibrium with the open
chain form. As indicated at the bottom, many such bifunctional
molecules (Structure 6) were investigated and many of the resultant compounds display salidiuretic effects.

Scheme III

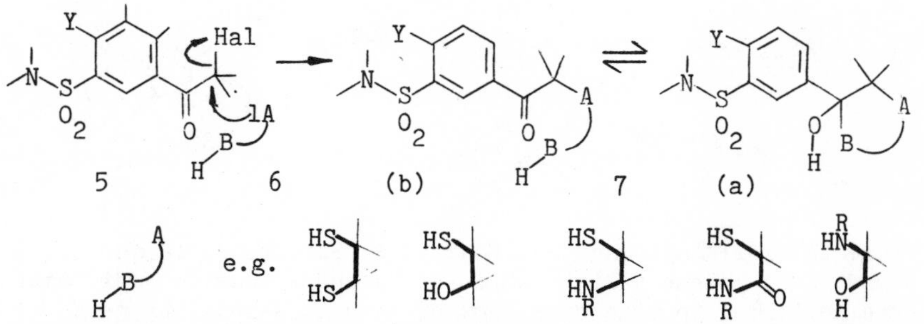

Thioureas (Structure 9) were used as the bifunctional molecules reacting as expected (11, 12) with the α-haloacetophenone
(Structure 8) to give isothiouronium salts (Structure 10b) (Scheme
IV). These compounds undergo cyclotautomerization to give thia-
zolidinol salts (Structure 10a). Treatment of these salts with
weak bases such as triethylamine or sodium bicarbonate affords the
free bases (Structure 11).

Scheme IV

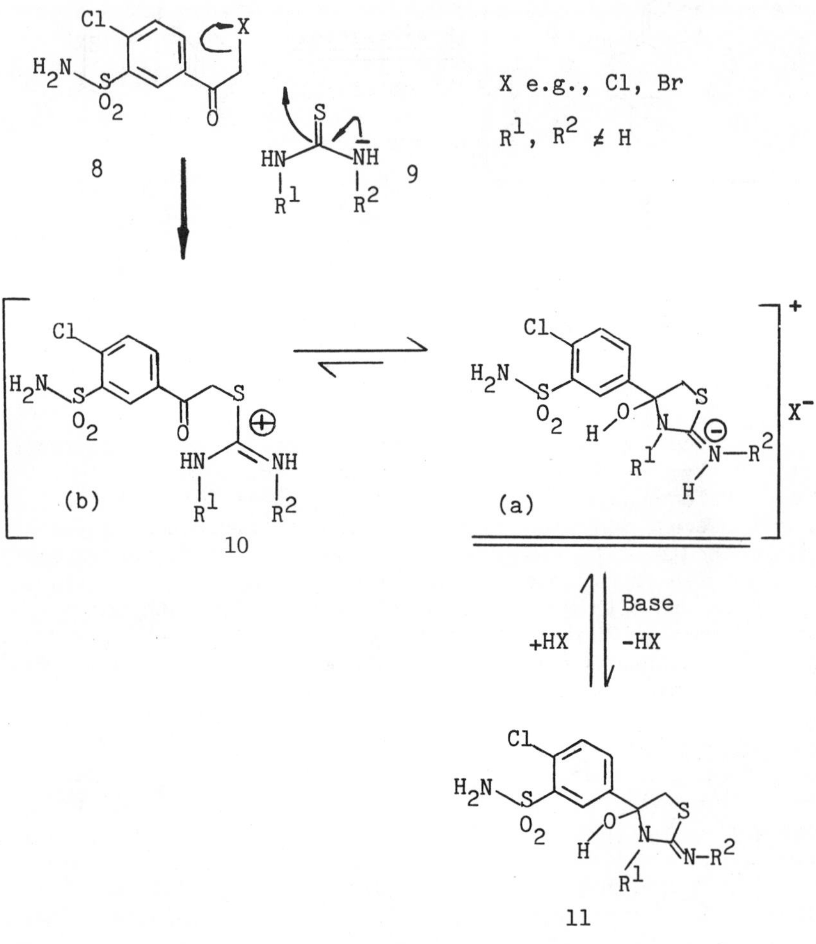

These thiazolidinylbenzenesulfonamides (Structures 10 and 11) were found to be potent salidiuretic agents and extensive modifications were performed to elucidate further structure-activity relationships. The following comments with respect to structure-activity relationships pertain to studies with rats.

Structure 12a of Scheme V shows where modifications may be made.

Scheme V

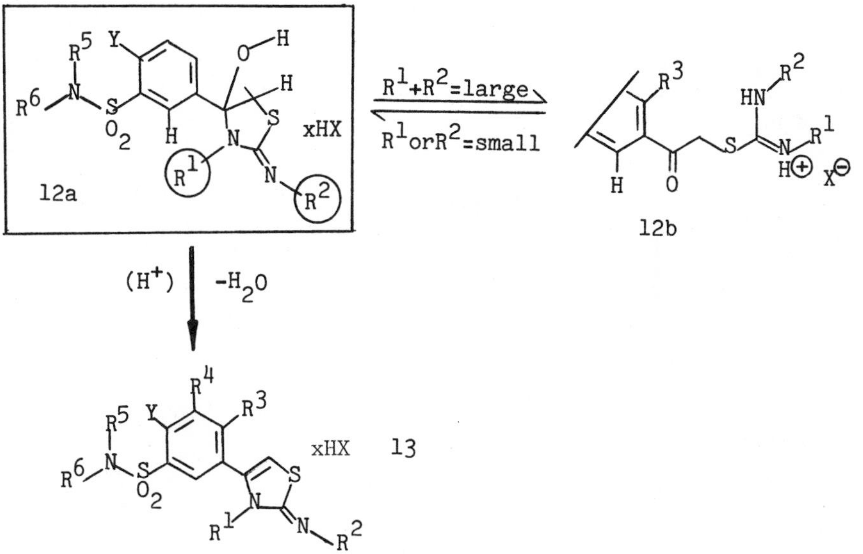

As mentioned above, there is a tautomeric equilibrium between the thiazolidine and the open chain isothiourea forms (Structures 12a and 12b). This equilibrium could be proved in related structural systems by IR and NMR spectroscopic studies (11). The equilibrium is easily observed in the IR spectrum by examining the intensity of the carbonyl band near 1680 cm^{-1}, which is caused only by the open chain form. When both R^1 and R^2 are rather bulky substituents, such as cyclohexyl, cyclooctyl and cyclododecyl, there may be a carbonyl absorption at 1680 cm^{-1} suggesting a greater contribution of the open chain form. In the case where R^1 and R^2 are cyclododecyl, there is a marked reduction in salidiuretic activity. This reduced activity appears to be due more to the overall increased bulk of the molecule than just to its existing in the open chain form (Structure 12b). Optimal salidiuretic activity is associated with compounds where R^1 is a small substituent, such as methyl or ethyl, and R^2 is methyl, ethyl or even a bulkier substituent, such as cyclohexyl, cyclooctyl, benzyl, etc. Dehydration of the thiazolidines to thiazolines (Structure 13) is readily achieved by boiling with acetic acid. These compounds show reduced salidiuretic activity when compared to the corresponding thiazolidines (Structure 12).

Replacement of one or both sulfamoyl hydrogen atoms produces a decrease or a loss of salidiuretic activity in most of the known sulfamoyl diuretics. We were quite surprised to observe almost no decrease in salidiuretic activity when one of the sulfamoyl hydrogen atoms in formula 10 or 11 was replaced with alkyl groups, for example, with methyl to n-hexyl groups.

Furthermore, almost no decrease in activity was observed by
similar replacement of one hydrogen atom (R^5 or R^6) of formula 12
with phenyl, carbamoyl, acetyl or aralkyl groups, such as benzyl
or a substituted benzyl group.

Good salidiuretic activity but a slightly enhanced toxicity
was observed when both hydrogen atoms of the sulfamoyl group were
replaced, for example, with methyls or with methyl and benzyl
groups.

At this point we also tried to answer two other questions
with respect to structure-activity relationships. First, is the
sulfamoyl group necessary for salidiuretic activity?   A literature survey revealed compounds of general structure 14 where X or
Y are not a sulfamoyl group were reported by Manning and Houlihan
(12).

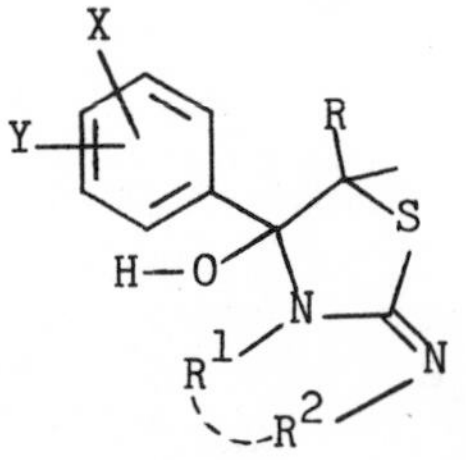

14

A salidiuretic activity is associated with these compounds;
however, compounds 12a containing a sulfamoyl group are much more
potent as salidiuretic agents. The second question was whether or
not the chlorine atom and sulfamoyl group could be interchanged.
The isomer 15 of tizolemide (Compound 16, Hoe 740) was synthesized
and was found to be almost devoid of salidiuretic activity.

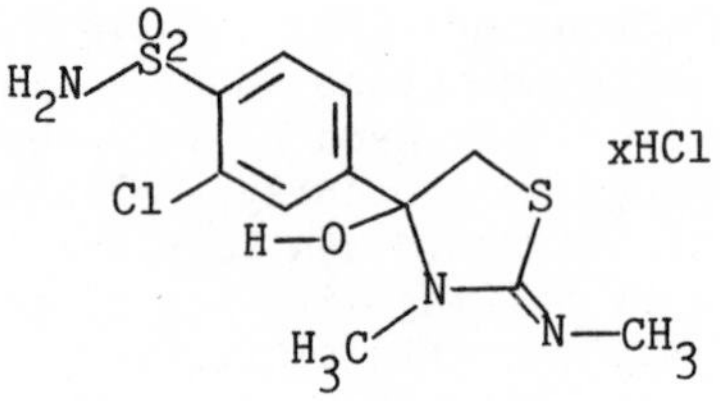

15

Optimal activity appears to be associated with the unsubstituted sulfamoyl group, so tizolemide was selected for further investigations.

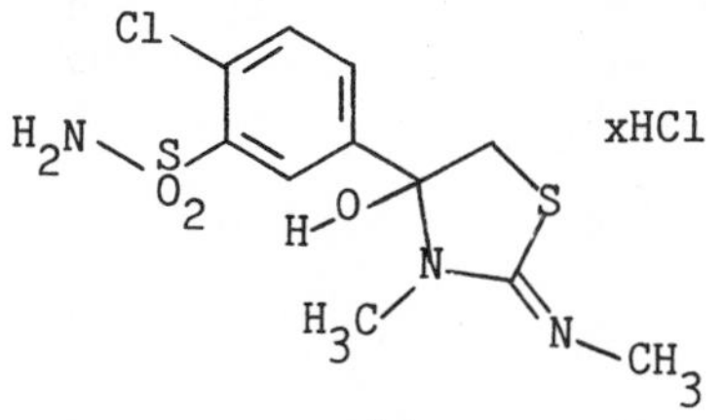

16
Tizolemide
(Hoe 740)

The hydrochloride salt is an odorless, colorless, crystalline, substance which is moderately soluble in water. Most other sulfonamide diuretics have an acidic or neutral function at the position meta to the sulfamoyl group. In contrast, tizolemide bears a basic substituent at this position.

Tizolemide was compared with hydrochlorothiazide and chlorthalidone in various pharmacological assays. On the following figures the abbreviations Hoe 740, HCT and Ch-on appear to indicate these agents.

ION EXCRETION IN RATS

Figure 1 shows the dose-response curves in rats after oral administration of tizolemide, hydrochlorothiazide and chlorthalidone. Only sodium excretion is shown, since excretion of chloride and water follow in a parallel manner. The curves are generally flat over a dose range of 0.25 to 32 mg/kg which is typical for thiazide-like diuretics. However, at higher dosages, Hoe 740 exerts an additional effect on the excretion of sodium, chloride and water. Micropuncture studies in rats revealed that the most intensive inhibition of sodium-reabsorption by Hoe 740 is located in the distal tubule. A slight activity was also observed in the loop of Henle which might account for the high-ceiling behavior of Hoe 740.

ION EXCRETION IN DOGS

Figure 2 shows the dose-response curves with respect to the sodium and chloride excretion in dogs after oral administration of tizolemide, hydrochlorothiazide and chlorthalidone. In contrast to the previous results with rats, these agents are much more potent in dogs. The curves are nearly identical. There was no significant difference between these agents in dogs over the dose range investigated.

30

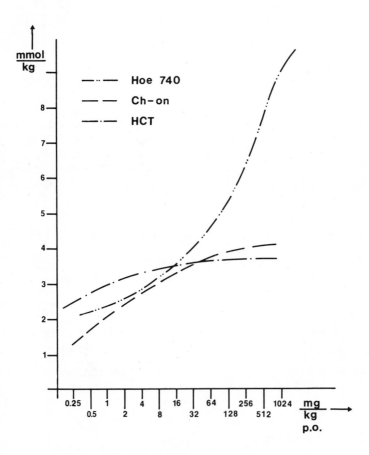

Figure 1.   Sodium excretion, rat, 5 hr

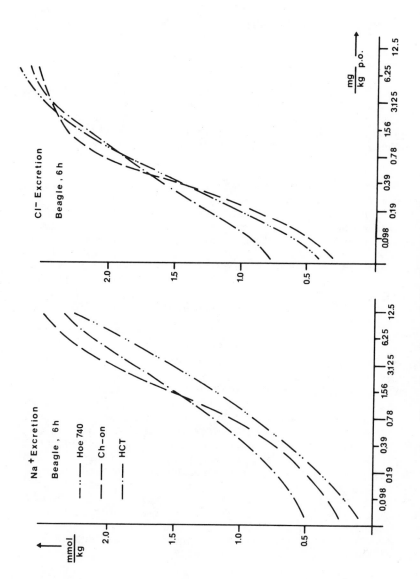

Figure 2. Sodium and chloride excretion, dog, 6 hr

THE ION RATIO

It is thought that a good diuretic agent should cause little or no enhanced excretion of potassium. It has been suggested that there is in many cases a close connection between the bicarbonate excretion and the excretion of potassium after treatment with diuretics (13, 14). Figure 3 shows the ratio of $Cl^-/Na^+ + K^+$ in dogs for Hoe 740, hydrochlorothiazide and chlorthalidone, produced in the previous experiment (Figure 2) over the saluretic active dose range. In the theoretical case where no other ions are excreted, this ratio would be equal to 1. If bicarbonate is also excreted, the ratio is less than 1. Figure 3 shows a higher $Cl^-/Na^+ + K^+$ ratio for Hoe 740 than for hydrochlorothiazide and chlorthalidone. This observation suggests that Hoe 740 would induce a lower excretion of potassium than chlorthalidone.

SODIUM AND POTASSIUM EXCRETION

Figure 4 shows the correlation between sodium and potassium excretion in dogs after i.v. administration of 12.5 mg/kg/h of chlorthalidone and Hoe 740. In comparison to the control group, there was a significant increase in sodium excretion after administration of both compounds. Chlorthalidone also causes a significant increase in potassium excretion, while potassium excretion after Hoe 740 is not significantly increased in comparison to the control group. This observation is presumably consistent with the higher $Cl^-/Na^+ + K^+$ ratio mentioned above for Hoe 740.

ANTIHYPERTENSIVE EFFECTS

Figure 5 shows the antihypertensive effects in rats treated with glycyrrhetinic acid after a daily administration of 50 mg/kg (p.o.) of Hoe 740, hydrochlorothiazide and chlorthalidone.
The glycyrrhetinic rat is a modified DOCA rat, as developed by Prof. Dr. Lindner (Hoechst AG) by use of glycyrrhetinic acid in place of 11-desoxycorticosteron-21-acetate. The high blood pressure is produced after a control period by treatment with Tyrode-solution as the drinking water and glycyrrhetinic acid (10 mg/kg daily). When a constant hypertension was achieved, the salidiuretic agent was administered while treatment with glycyrrhetinic acid was continued. The blood pressure was significantly decreased after Hoe 740, as well as, after treatment with the other two agents. When salidiuretic treatment was withdrawn, the blood pressure increased again but the previous hypertensive level was not achieved.

SERUM URIC ACID CONCENTRATIONS

Subchronic studies of the effects of Hoe 740 on serum uric acid concentrations have also been performed. Serum uric acid

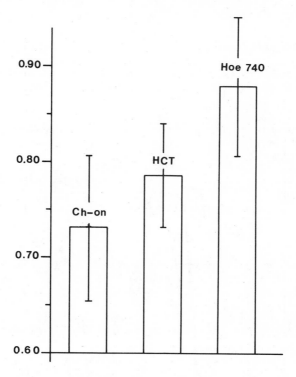

Figure 3.   Cl⁻/Na⁺ + K⁺, dog

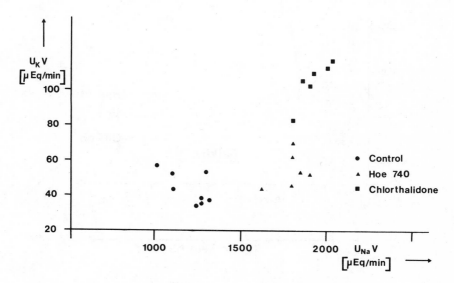

Figure 4.   Correlation between Na⁺ and K⁺ excretion, dog

34

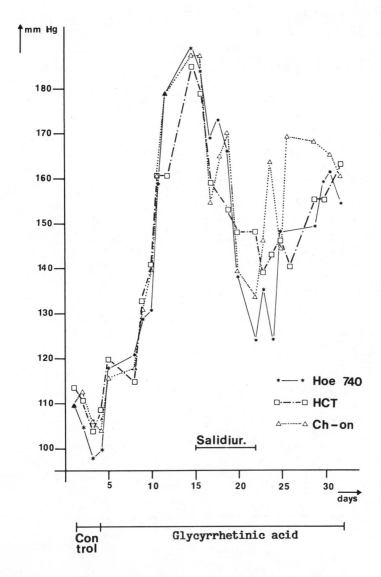

Figure 5. Antihypertensive effect in glycyrrhetinic rat

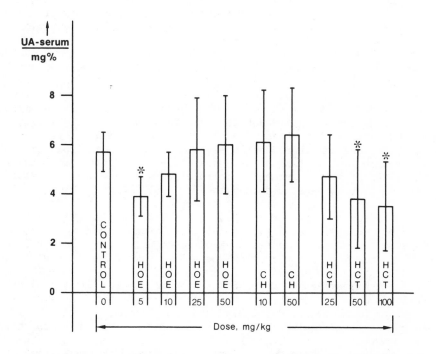

Figure 6.   Effect of Hoe 740 on UA-serum concentration in comparison with chlorthalidone and hydrochlorothiazide in oxonic rat

concentrations have also been performed. Serum uric acid levels
in dogs during 30 days treatment with 2.5, 8 and 25 mg/kg of Hoe
740 were not influenced; however, these levels were decreased in
normal rats during the same length of treatment after oral administration of Hoe 740 at 4, 40 and 400 mg/kg.

The effect of Hoe 740 on serum uric acid was also studied in
the oxonic rat (15, 16). Most mammals with the exception of some
primates and humans convert uric acid into allantoin by means of
the enzyme uricase. Allantoin is readily excreted in the urine
because of its water solubility and its poor reabsorption in the
kidney. Treatment of rats with the potassium salt of oxonic acid
inhibits uricase and results in elevated serum uric acid levels.
These hyperuricemic rats are treated once a day for three days
with the test substance as well as oxonic acid. At the end of the
test period, the animals are sacrificed and serum levels of uric
acid are determined. Figure 6 shows the results with the oxonic
rat. In this test, chlorthalidone produced at most a very slight
increase in serum uric acid levels. Hydrochlorothiazide in higher
doses produced a significant decrease in serum uric acid levels.
In contrast, at low doses, Hoe 740 displayed an antihyperuricemic
activity, whereas at doses higher than 10 mg/kg, no significant
difference from control animals was observed. Hoe 740 is being
investigated at the present time to elucidate the possible mechanism of this dose-related behavior.

Of special importance is that decreased serum uric acid
levels after 10 mg/kg of Hoe 740 (p.o.) could be demonstrated also
in Cebus monkeys (cebus albifrons) whose metabolism of uric acid
is similar to man. The decrease of serum uric acid concentration
was significant ($p < 0.05$) after Hoe 740 in comparison to the
control group.

Acknowledgments - We wish to thank Dr. Cragoe for the oppor-
tunity to present our work with these thiazolidines. We also wish
to thank Dr. Lochelt, Dr. Schutz and Prof. Kramer for their
subchronic studies in rats and dogs. Furthermore, I wish to thank
my co-workers, Miss Ansuhn, Mrs. Fischer and Mr. Ahlborn. I wish
to thank Dr. Lawrence Martin for his assistance in the English
translation.

                     Literature Cited
1. Saxl, P. and Heilig, R., Wien. Klin. Wschr. (1920), 33, 943.
2. Vogl, A., Amer. Heart J. (1950), 39, 881.
3. Hoechst, DRP. (1925) 423031; Friedlander 15, 1608.
4. American Cyanamid, U.S. Pat. 2554816 (1951).
5. Novello, F. C. and Sprague, J. M., J. Amer. Chem. Soc.
(1957), 79, 2028.
6. Ciba, Brit. Pat. (1960), 847064.
7. Sturm, K., Siedel, W., Weyer, R. and Ruschig, H., Ber.
Deut. Chem. Ges. (1966), 99, 328.
8. Schultz, E. M., Cragoe, E. J., Jr., Bicking, J. B., Bolhofer,
W. A., Sprague, J. M., J. Med. Pharm. Chem. (1962), 5, 660.
9. Merkel, W., Bormann, D., Mania, D., Muschaweck, R. and

Hropot, M., Eur. J. Med. Chem.-Chim. Ther. (1976), 11, 399.
10. Graf, W., Girod, E., Schmid, E. and Stoll, W. G., Helv. Chim. Acta (1959), 42, 1085.
11. Sharpe, C. J., Shadbolt, R. S., Ashford, A. and Ross, J. W., J. Med. Chem. (1971), 14, 977.
12. Houlihan, W. J. and Manning, R. E., U.S. Pat.. 3,671,533.
13. Muschaweck, R., "Atti del Symposium Internazionale sul Potassio in Biologia ed in Medicina," Siena, May 22-23 (1965).
14. Meng, K. and Loew, D., "Diuretika: Chemie, Pharmakologie, Therapie," 184, Georg Thieme Verlag, Stuttgart (1974).
15. Musil, J. and Sandow, J., "Amino Acid Transport and Uric Acid Transport," Eds. Silbernagl, S., Lang, F. and Greger, R., 227, Georg Thieme Verlag, Stuttgart (1975).
16. Musil, J., "Second International Symposium on Purine Metabolism in Man," Eds. Mathias M. Muller, Erich Kaiser and J. Edwin Seegmiller, 179, Baden, Austria (1976).

RECEIVED August 21, 1978.

4

Sulfonamide Diuretics

L. H. WERNER, E. HABICHT, and J. ZERGENYI

Research Department, Pharmaceuticals Division, CIBA–GEIGY Corp., Summit, NJ 07901 and Research Department, Pharmaceuticals Division, CIBA–GEIGY Ltd., Basle, Switzerland

More than twenty years have passed since the discovery of the thiazide diuretics. Since then many new developments in this field have occurred. The discovery of the thiazide diuretics in 1957-58 was the beginning of a new era in the treatment of edema and hypertension. Prior to the introduction of the thiazide diuretics, one had to rely on the mercurial diuretics and later, on the carbonic anhydrase inhibitors with their well known drawbacks. The carbonic anhydrase inhibitors acted mainly in the proximal tubule leading to increased urinary excretion of Na^+, K^+, and HCO_3^- and, as a consequence, to metabolic acidosis. At the time the carbonic anhydrase inhibitors were being developed, it was, however, the firm conviction of Drs. Beyer ([1]) and Baer of Merck Sharp and Dohme that a sulfonamide diuretic could be found that was saluretic, i.e., that increased urinary Na^+ and Cl^- excretion in equivalent quantities and therefore would not produce metabolic acidosis, if it worked at the appropriate site along the nephron. This working hypothesis eventually led to chlorothiazide.

It is now known that, depending on the site of action in the nephron, different diuretic profiles can be obtained, ranging from the carbonic anhydrase inhibitors to the thiazides and high-ceiling diuretics as is shown in Figure 1 ([2], [3]). Chemical structures, representing different types of diuretics have varied to a considerable extent.

The structures of these various classes of diuretics are exemplified by the carbonic anhydrase inhibitors, acetazolamide (4) and dichlorphenamide (5), the thiazide saluretic, chloro-thiazide (6), the high-ceiling diuretics, furosemide (7), etha-crynic acid (8) and bumetanide (9), the uricosuric diuretic, tienilic acid (10), and the more recent compounds, muzolimine (11) and MK-447 (12), the last two representing compounds without a sulfonamide or carboxy group (Figure 2).

Some of the work that was carried out in our laboratories in the area of sulfonamide diuretics will be presented. The sulfonamide diuretics currently in use are effective and safe;

0-8412-0464-0/78/47-083-**038**$05.00/0

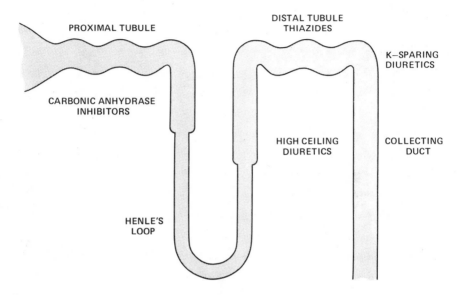

PROXIMAL TUBULE

DISTAL TUBULE
THIAZIDES

K−SPARING
DIURETICS

CARBONIC ANHYDRASE
INHIBITORS

HIGH CEILING
DIURETICS

COLLECTING
DUCT

HENLE'S
LOOP

Figure 1.   Representation of sites of action of diuretics in the nephron

TABLE I

Diuretic Screen

Reference Compounds	Unanesthetized Dog
Hydrochlorothiazide 5.0 mg/kg p.o.	1300 μEq Na/kg/210 min.
Furosemide 5./0 mg/kg p.o.	5200 μEq Na/kg/210 min.
Bumetanide 0.3 mg/kg p.o.	5700 μEq Na/kg/210 min.

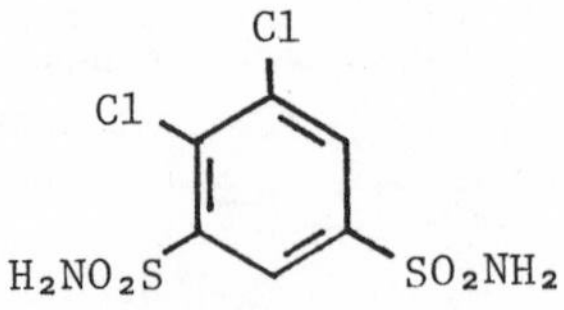

dichlorphenamide

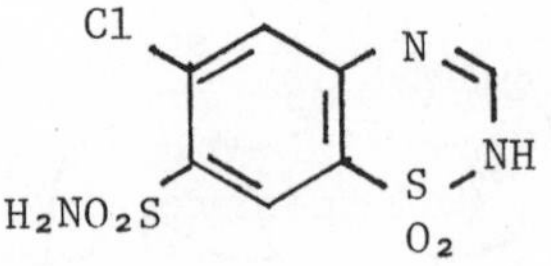

chlorothiazide

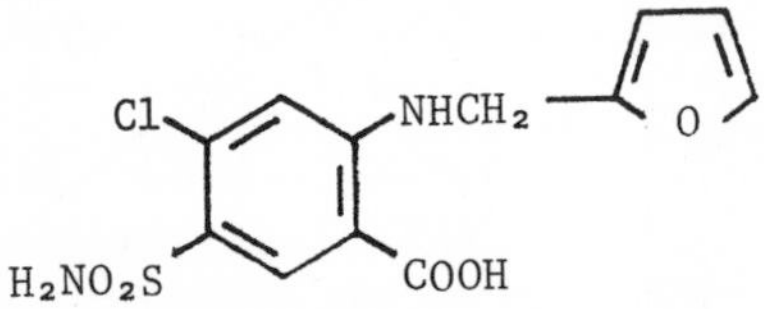

furosemide

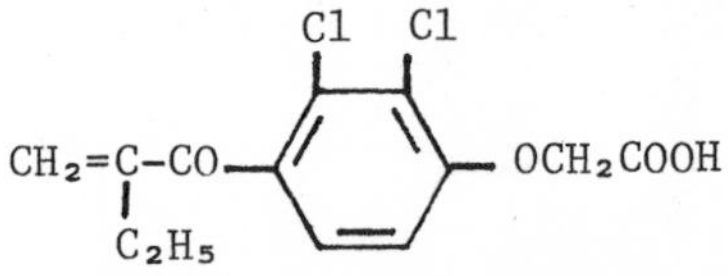

ethacrynic acid

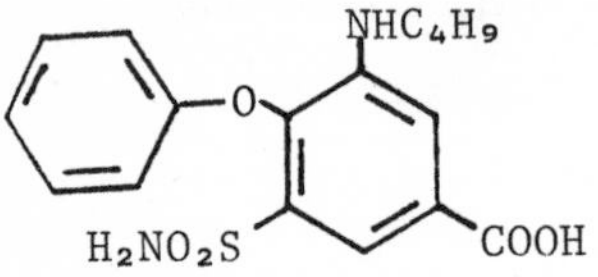

bumetanide

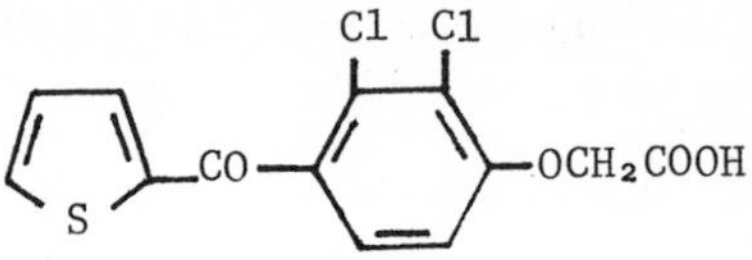

tienilic acid

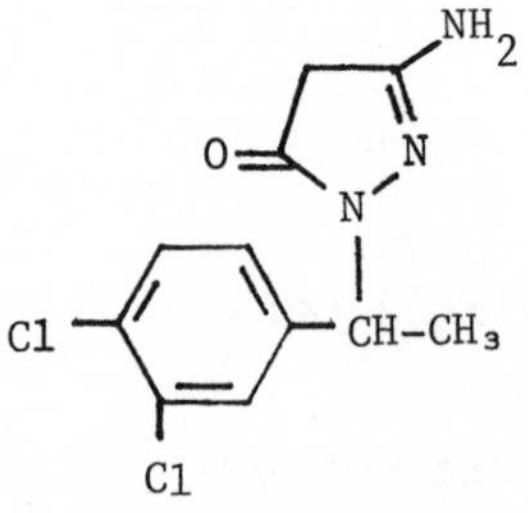

muzolimine

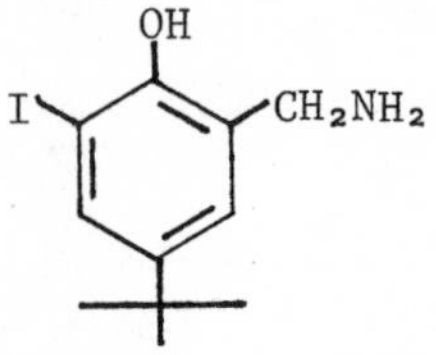

MK 447

Figure 2.   Various classes of diuretics

there are, however, three undesirable side effects associated
with the chronic administration of these compounds: (1) potassium depletion, (2) elevation of serum uric acid and (3) hyperglycemia. In patients with a normal fasting blood sugar, it
would appear that the risk of precipitating diabetes is small.
In patients who already have diabetes, the chance of disturbing
the control of blood sugar is substantial. We hoped that our work
would provide compounds either with less effect on potassium
excretion or on blood glucose levels.

The compounds prepared were tested in rats and dogs;
however, only results in dogs are reported as an indication of
the relative potency of these compounds. Table I shows the
values obtained with three standard sulfonamide diuretics in our
diuretic screening using unanesthetized dogs. The values shown
in Figures 3 to 7 also represent μEq Na/kg/210 min.

In our first approach we decided to study bi- and tricyclic
compounds derived from intermediates which had yielded highly
active diuretics.

Initially, we studied compounds derived from the 2-hydra-
zino-5-sulfamoylbenzoic acid (Compound 1) previously described by
Sturm and co-workers (7) (Figure 3). The hydrazone (Compound 2)
derived from phenylacetaldehyde, was only slightly active.
Hydrazines such as compound 3 obtained by catalytic reduction of
the corresponding hydrazone were moderately active at 5 mg/kg in
the dog. On refluxing in dilute HCl, the hydrazine (Compound 3)
cyclized to the indazolone (Compound 5), which was almost inactive. Fischer indole ring closure of the hydrazone (Compound 2)
in acetic acid yielded the indole (Compound 4) which exhibited
diuretic activity at 50 mg/kg. All compounds were administered
orally.

Reaction of the 2-hydrazino-5-sulfamoylbenzoic acid (Compound 1) with cyclohexanone (Figure 3) followed by cyclization
yielded the tetrahydrocarbazole (Compound 6) which was subsequently reduced catalytically in trifluoroacetic acid with
platinum to the hexahydrocarbazole (Compound 7). Both compounds
6 and 7 had moderate diuretic activity at 100 mg and 50 mg/kg in
the dog.

Another approach started with 2,4-dichloro-3-nitro-5-
sulfamoylbenzoic acid (Compound 8, Figure 4). Treatment of
compound 8 with sodium hydroxide yielded the salicylic acid
derivative (Compound 9) (13). Reduction of the nitro group in
compound 9 followed by fusion with butyric anhydride or benzoic
anhydride gave the benzoxazoles (Compounds 10a and 10b, respectively). Only the 2-phenyl derivative (Compound 10b) showed
appreciable activity at 20 mg/kg in the dog.

Similarly, the benzimidazole (Compound 12, Figure 4) was
prepared. It was inactive. Starting with the 3-amino-4-
anilino-5-sulfamoylbenzoic acid (Compounds 13a (9) and 13b), two
other benzimidazoles (Compounds 14a and 14b, Figure 4) were
prepared, but were also inactive as diuretics.

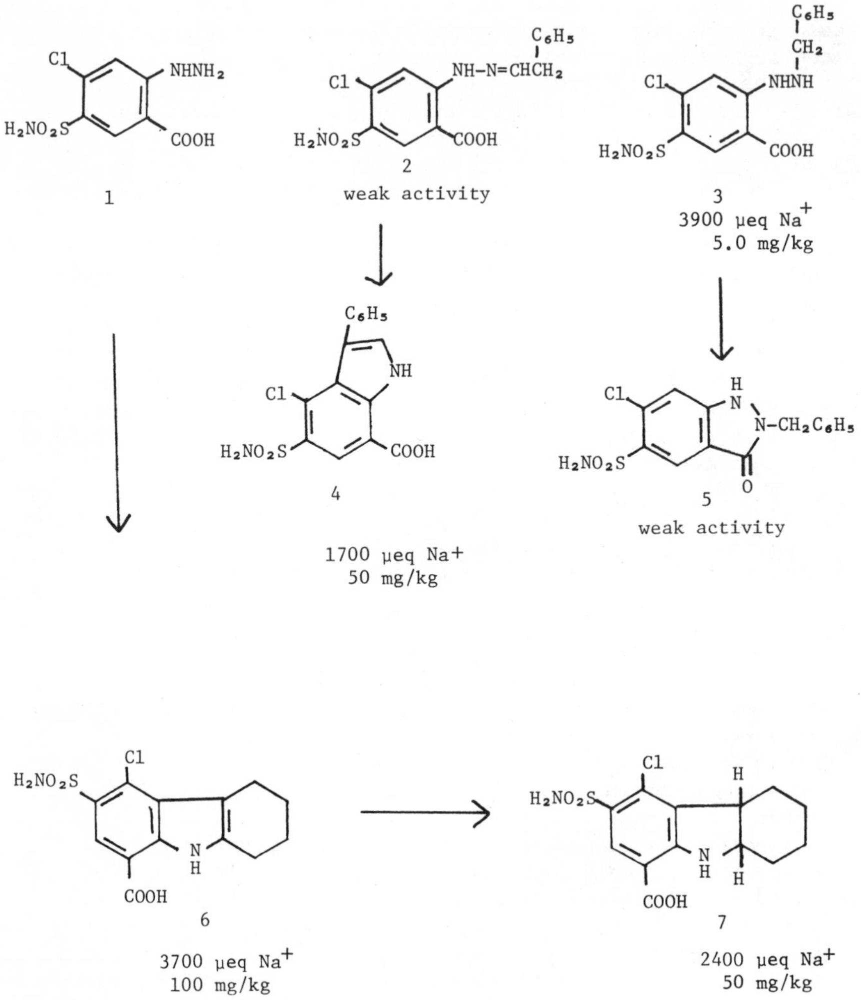

Figure 3.   Compounds derived from the 2-hydrazino-5-sulfamoylbenzoic acid

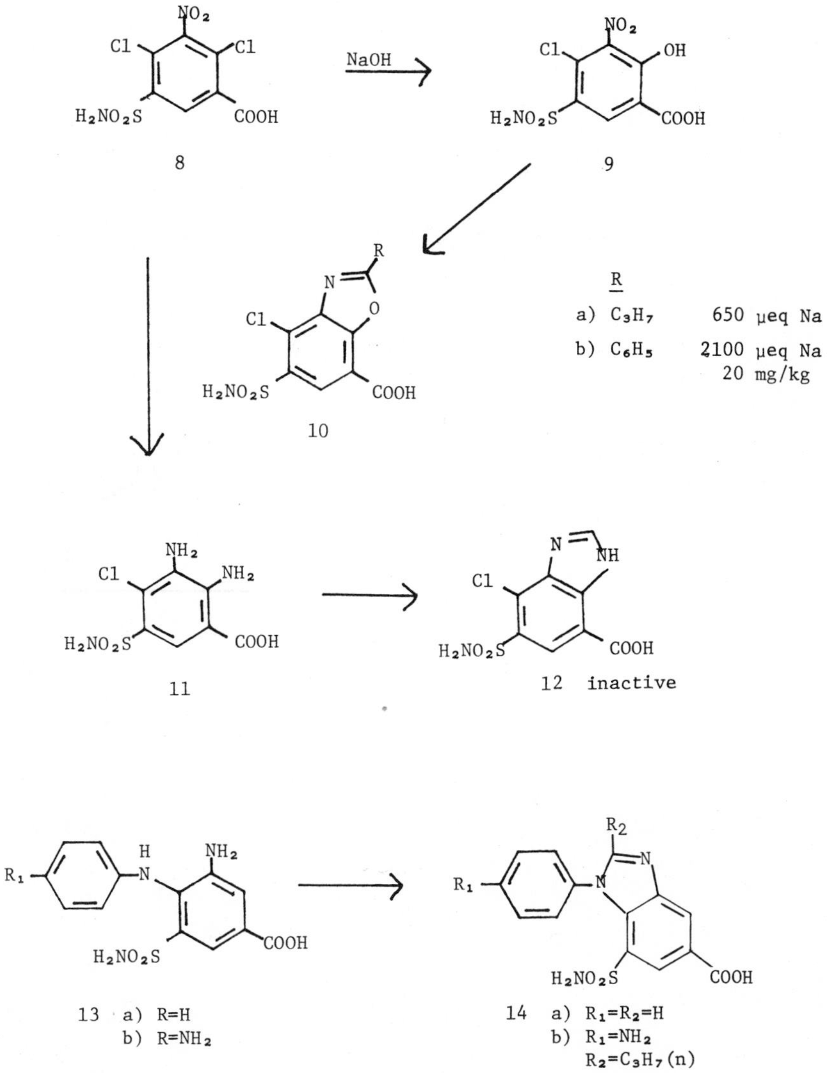

Figure 4. Benzoxazole and benzimidazole derivatives

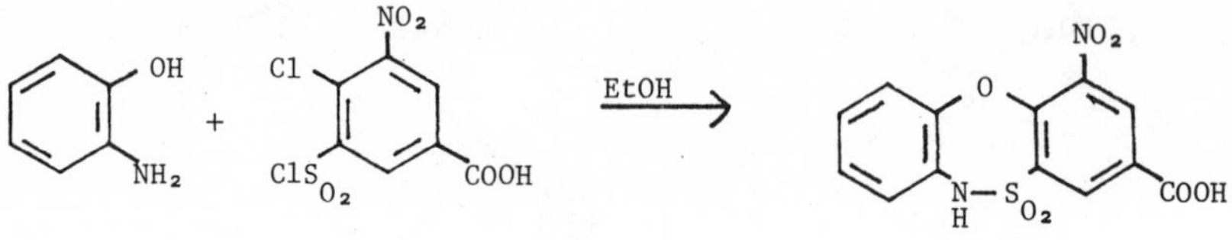

Figure 5.   Tricyclic derivatives

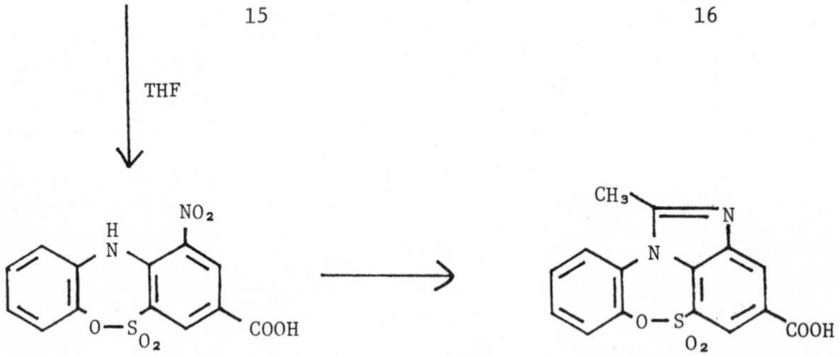

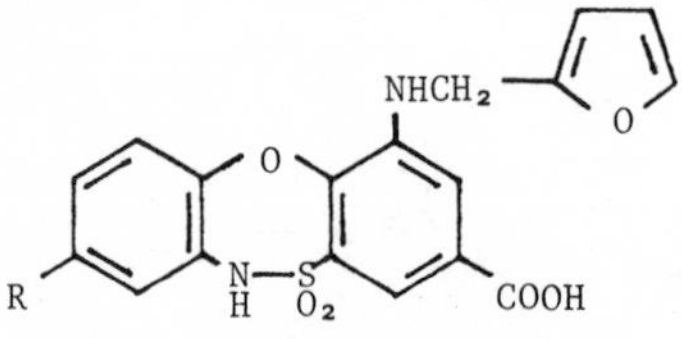

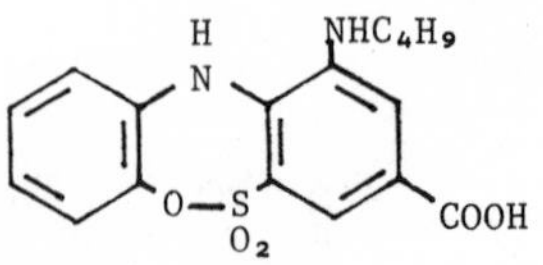

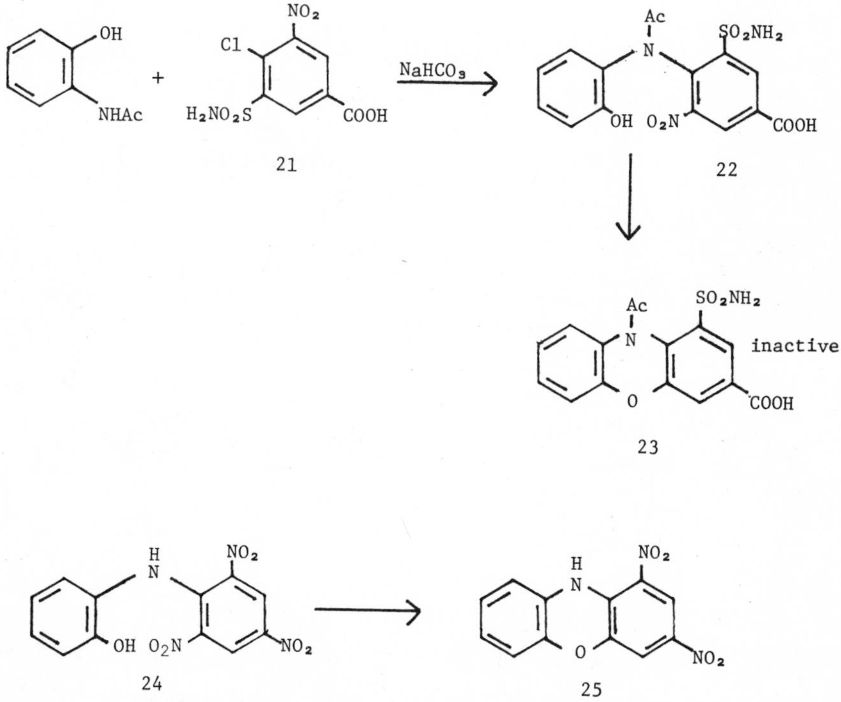

Figure 6. Phenoxazines and phenothiazines

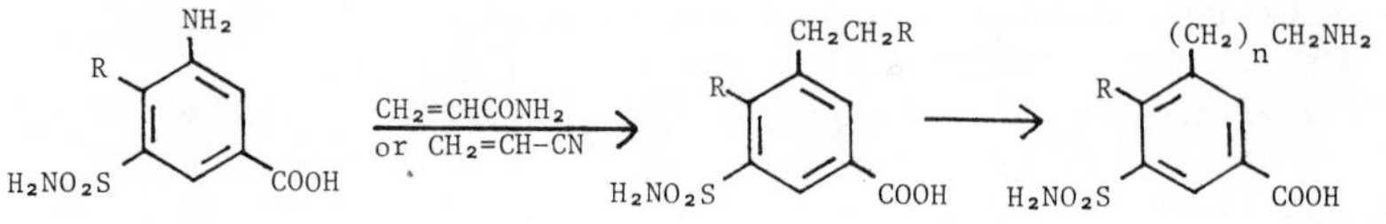

26 a) R=Cl
b) R=OC_6H_5

27 a) R= $CONH_2$
b) R= CN

28 a) n=1 } R=Cl, OC_6H_5
b) n=2 }

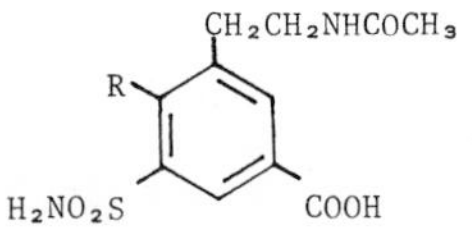

29 R= Cl, OC_6H_5

inactive

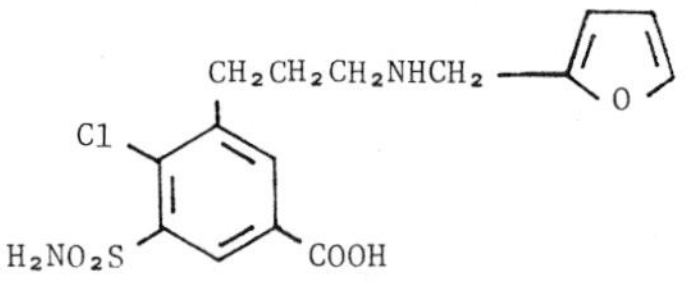

30

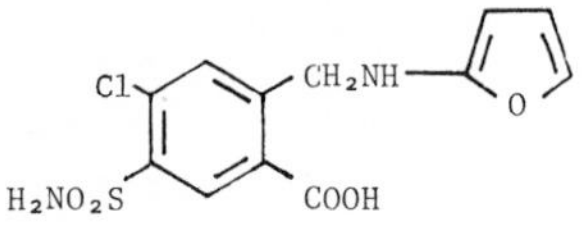

31

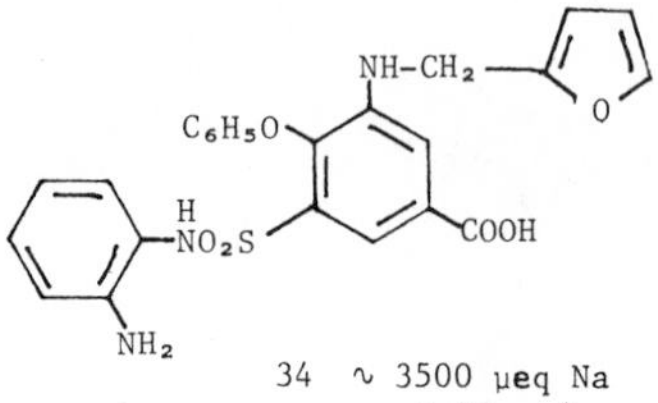

34 ∿ 3500 μeq Na
1.25 mg/kg

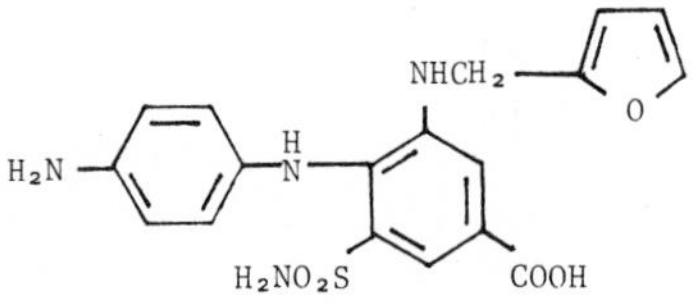

35 ∿ 6000 μeq Na
1.25 mg/kg

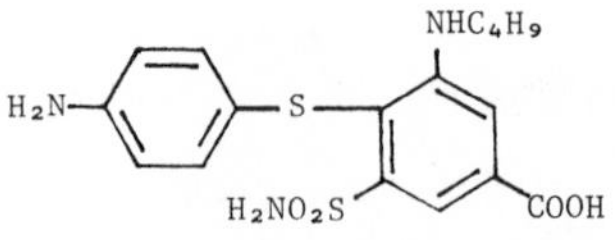

36 ∿ 6000 μeq Na
1.25 mg/kg

Figure 7. Monocyclic aromatic sulfonamide derivatives

Tricyclic derivatives, as shown in Figure 5, were also investigated. The reaction of o-aminophenol with 4-chloro-5-chlorosulfonyl-3-nitro-benzoic acid (Compound 15) (14) was of interest. Depending on the solvent, ethanol or THF, sulfonylation occurred on oxygen or nitrogen. Ring closure of the sulfonamide intermediate in aqueous NaHCO$_3$ yielded compound 16, whereas the sulfonyloxy intermediate ring closed directly to yield the isomeric tricyclic compound 17 (Figure 5).

The structure of compound 17 was confirmed by reduction of the nitro group to the amine and ring closure to the imidazole derivative (Compound 18) by refluxing in acetic anhydride.

Several derivatives of these two tricyclic compounds were prepared, for example, compounds 19 and 20, both were inactive as diuretics (Figure 5).

Reaction of o-acetaminophenol in aqueous NaHCO$_3$ solution with the sulfamoylbenzoic acid (Compound 21) (14) gave the N-acetyldiphenylamine derivative (Compound 22) in low yield (Figure 6). Whether this compound arises by direct reaction of the highly reactive chlorosulfamoylbenzoic acid (Compound 21) with the acetamino group of the phenol or is formed via a Smiles rearrangement of an intermediate diphenyl ether has not been explored. The main reaction product was the phenoxazine (Compound 23). Similar ring closure reactions via a Smiles rearrangement to phenoxazines and phenothiazines, e.g., compound 24 to compound 25, have been reviewed by Truce, et al (15). The phenoxazine (Compound 23) as well as the deacetylated derivative had no diuretic activity.

Certain monocyclic aromatic sulfonamide derivatives were also studied. Starting with the 3-amino-5-sulfamoylbenzoic acid (Compound 26, Figure 7) (9, 14), the amino group was replaced by a propionamide or propionitrile group under conditions of a Meerwein reaction (Compound 16) using acrylamide or acrylonitrile, respectively, to yield compounds 27a and 27b. A Hoffmann degradation of compound 27a gave the aminoethyl derivative (Compound 28a). Reduction of the nitrile (Compound 27b) yielded the aminopropyl derivative (Compound 28b, Figure 7). The N-acetyl derivative (Compound 29) was inactive. The effect of inserting a three carbon chain in the 3-position of the sulfamoylbenzoic acid moiety of the bumetanide-type diuretics was studied. Compound 30, which is related to bumetanide, was only weakly active, as was compound 31, which differs from furosemide only by a CH$_2$ group (Figure 7). This may be related to the increased basicity of the benzylic amine function. Feit and co-workers have shown that the aromatic amino group in bumetanide can be replaced by an O- or S- ether linkage without a pronounced change in diuretic potency; however, in the anthranilic acid (furosemide) series, the structural requirements are more stringent.

It is generally accepted that substitution on the sulfonamide nitrogen of sulfonamide diuretics lowers the diuretic

TABLE II

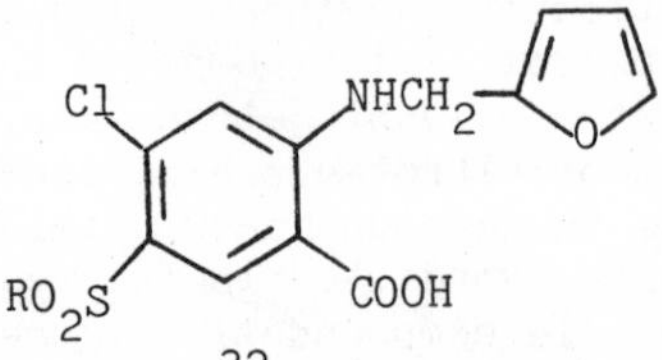

32

	R	Dose mg/kg p.o.	μEq/kg/4 hr Na$^+$	K$^+$	Ref.
a:	NH$_2$	6.25	5000	935	(Furosemide)
b:	NHCH$_3$	5	slight activity		
c:	NHCH$_2$C$_6$H$_5$	5	1000		
d:	NHC$_6$H$_5$	6.25	2200	400	(18)
	Control		370	340	

TABLE III

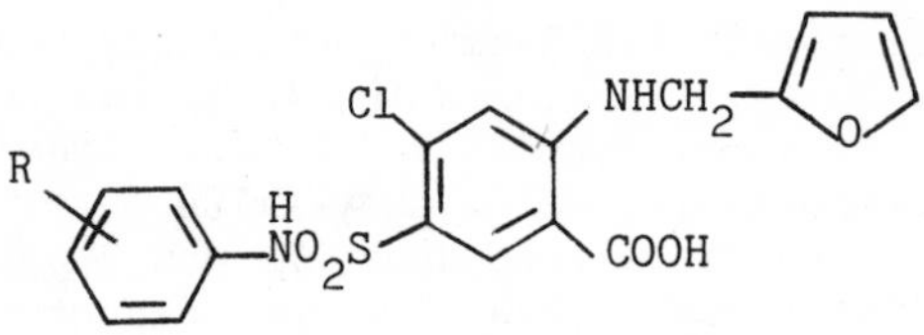

33

	R	Dose mg/kg p.o.	μEq/kg/4 hr Na$^+$	K$^+$	Ref.
a:	p-Cl	5	very slight activity		
b:	p-NH$_2$	5	5000	800	(18)
c:	p-NH-CH$_3$	5	slight activity		
d:	p-N(CH$_3$)$_2$	5	inactive		
e:	o-NH$_2$	2.5	5500	900	(18)
	Control		370	340	

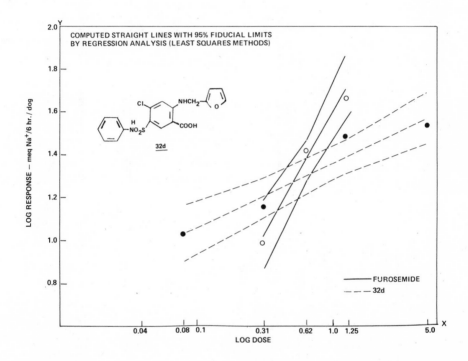

Figure 8. Comparative dose response curves—furosemide vs. compound 32d—Na⁺ excretion in dogs

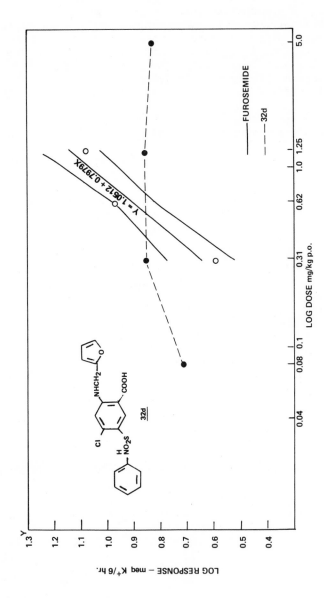

Figure 9. Comparative dose response curves—furosemide vs. compound 32d—K⁺ excretion in dogs

activity. Since we were not primarily looking for enhanced
potency but were interested in trying to modify some of the other
properties such as potassium depletion and effects on blood
glucose levels, we investigated this area.

Compound 32a (Table II) is furosemide, methylation of the
sulfamoyl nitrogen as in compound 32b drastically reduced the
diuretic activity, the N-benzyl derivative (Compound 32c) re-
tained a modest degree of activity. Surprisingly, the N-phenyl
derivative (Compound 32d) was quite natriuretic and appeared to
have very little effect on potassium excretion as shown in Table
II.

This observation was further explored by introducing a
substituent on the phenyl ring attached to the sulfamoyl group of
compound 32a. The p-chlorophenyl derivative (Compound 33a, Table
III) was only weakly active; however, the p-aminophenyl derivative (Compound 33b) proved to be a very active diuretic. Methylation of the amino group as in compounds 33c and 33d greatly
reduced the activity; the 4-dimethylaminophenylsulfonamide
(Compound 33d) was actually inactive at the 5 mg/kg dose (Table
III).

The o-aminophenylsulfonamide derivative (Compound 33e) was
more active on a weight basis than the p-aminophenyl derivative
(Compound 33b). Unfortunately, potassium excretion was also
elevated.

The finding that a para- or ortho-aminophenyl group can
enhance activity was also applied to the 3-amino-5-sulfamoyl-
benzoic acid series (Figure 7). Compound 34 had moderate diuretic activity at 1.25 mg/kg p.o. in the dog. Both compounds 35
and 36 were active diuretics (19, 20). Compound 36 was of
somewhat greater interest and was active in a dose related sense
over a range of 0.02 mg to 1 mg/kg. Thus, a number of compounds
of potential interest had been found and considered worthy of
further study.

Compound 32d (Table II) was of interest because it appeared
to have very little effect on potassium excretion. It was an
active diuretic in dogs and reached a natriuretic ceiling at a
dose of approximately 6 mg/kg. Osmolar clearance increased
two-to three-fold, while reabsorption of solute free water
remained positive in the dog. Figure 8 shows the dose response
curve for sodium excretion in dogs. At higher dosages, sodium
excretion leveled off for compound 32d, whereas it continued
upward with furosemide. Figure 9 shows the effect on potassium
excretion, which was practically unaffected by higher doses.
Clinical trials in normal volunteers, however, failed to produce
any diuretic effects.

Compound 33b was also studied in greater detail. The
diuretic effects in the dog resembled those obtained with furosemide, except that at doses above 10 mg/kg, the excretion of
Na^+, Cl^-, K^+ and water decreased somewhat (Figure 10). During
peak diuresis, the urine was almost isotonic. Renal plasma flow

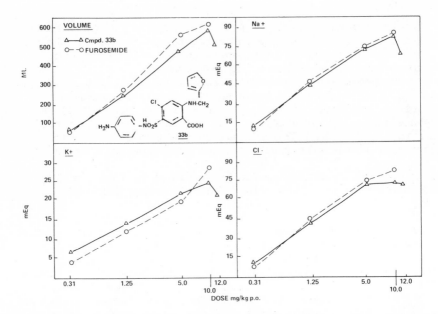

Figure 10. Diuretic effects of compound 33b and furosemide in dogs—excretion per dog per 6 hr

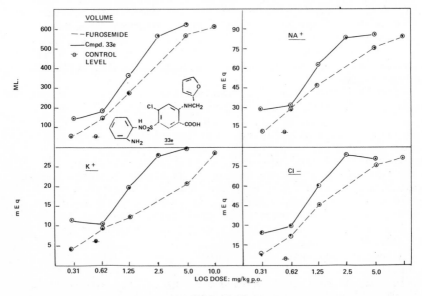

Figure 11. Diuretic effects of compound 33e and furosemide in dogs—excretion per dog per 6 hr

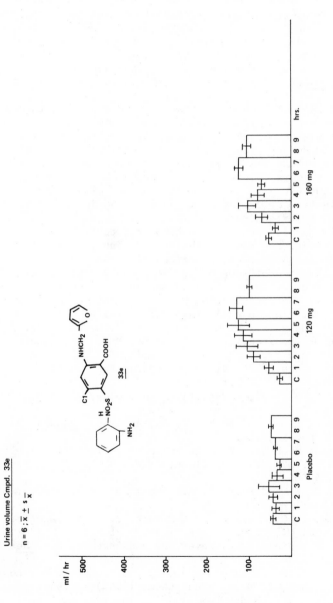

Figure 12. Diuretic response in normal volunteers

and glomerular filtration rate were only slightly affected.

In normal volunteers, doses of 40 to 120 mg produced a rapid onset of diuresis which persisted for 5 to 6 hours, similar to that of furosemide. The natriuretic effect reached a ceiling at the 80 to 120 mg dose and was about equal to 40 mg of furosemide.

Compound 33e was a somewhat more potent diuretic in dogs than furosemide. The onset of action was prompt, reaching a peak after 90 minutes and subsiding after 5 to 6 hours. The dose response curves for urine volume, Na^+, K^+ and Cl^- are shown in Figure 11.

In normal volunteers, contrary to the results obtained in animal experiments, compound 33e was not a high-ceiling diuretic. An activity plateau was reached at 80-120 mg, two to three times the threshold dosage (Figure 12). Its natriuretic effect at this level was less than that induced by 100 mg of hydrochlorothiazide. Interestingly, this compound did not produce a peak level of excretion, but rather a more constant effect persisting over five hours. This type of diuretic response may be desirable in the treatment of hypertension.

Unfortunately, none of the compounds described were potassium-sparing nor did they have appreciably less effect on glucose tolerance; however, no uricosuric effect was observed. This brief overview of some of our work on sulfonamide diuretics illustrates one of the problems we encounter in medicinal chemistry; namely, that encouraging biological data in animals do not always translate into equally favorable clinical results.

Acknowledgments – We wish to thank Dr. O. Büch, Dr. P. R. Hedwall and Dr. J. Kraetz, Basle, and Dr. M. J. Antonaccio, Dr. W. E. Barrett and Mr. R. Rutledge, Summit, for the pharma cological data and Dr. P. R. Imhof, Basle, for the clinical data.

Literature Cited

1.   Beyer, K. H., Jr., Perspectives in Biology and Med. (1976), 19, 500.

2.   Jacobson, H. R. and Kokko, J. P., Ann. Rev. Pharmacol. Toxicol. (1976), 16, 201.

3.   Anderton, J. L. and Kincaid-Smith, P., Drugs (1971), 1, 54.

4.   Roblin, R. O., Jr., and Clapp, J. W., J. Am. Chem. Soc. (1950), 72, 4890.

5.   Beyer, K. H. and Baer, J. E., Pharmacol. Rev. (1961), 13, 517.

6.   Novello, F. C., Bell, S. C., Abrams, E. L. A., Ziegler, C. and Sprague, J. M., J. Org. Chem. (1960), 25, 965.

7.   Sturm, K., Siedel, W., Weyer, R. and Ruschig, H., Chem. Ber. (1966), 99, 329.

8.   Schultz, E. M., Cragoe, E. J., Jr., Bicking, J. B., Bolhofer, W. A. and Sprague, J. M., J. Med. Chem. (1962), 5, 660.

9.   Feit, P. W., J. Med. Chem. (1971), 14, 432.

10. Thuillier, G., Laforest, J., Cariou, B. Bessin, P., Bonnet, J. and Thuillier, J., Eur. J. Med. Chem. (1974), 9, 625.

11. Möller, E., Horstmann, H., Meng, K. and Loew, D., Experientia

(1977), 33, 382.

12. Affrime, M. B., Lowenthal, D. T., Onesti, G. Busby, P.,
Swartz, C. and Lei, B., Clin. Pharmacol. Ther. (1977), 21, 97.

13. Liebenow, W., Canadian Patent 952,536 (1974), Chem. Abstr.
(1975), 82, P170,430.

14. Feit, P. W., Bruun, H. and Nielsen, C. K., J. Med Chem.
(1970), 13, 1071.

15. Truce, W. E., Kreider, E. M. and Brand, W. W., "Organic
Reactions", Vol. 18, p. 99, Ed., W. G. Dauben, John Wiley & Sons,
Inc., New York, 1970.

16. Müller, E., Angew. Chem. (1949), 61, 179.

17. Feit, P. W., Tvaermose-Nielsen, O. B. and Bruun, H., J. Med.
Chem. (1974), 17, 572.

18. Werner, L. H., U.S. Patent 3,812,104 (1974); Chem. Abstr.
(1969), 70, P67908r.

19. Werner, L. H., U.S. Patent 3,927,218 (1975); Chem. Abstr.
(1976), 84, P105217p.

20. Werner, L. H., U.S. Patent 3,939,267 (1976); Ger. Offen.
2,349,900 (1974).

RECEIVED August 21, 1978.

5

Diuretic and Uricosuric Properties of Tienilic Acid (Ticrynafen) in Mice, Rats, and Anesthetized Beagle Dogs
Antihypertensive Activity in SH Rats and Structure–Activity Relationship

P. BESSIN, J. BONNET, M. F. MALIN, C. JACQUEMIN, N. DE BREZE, I. PELAS, L. DESGROUX, B. AGIER, and M. DUTARTE

Albert Rolland Center for Research and Pharmacology (CREPHAR), 4, Rue de la Division Leclerc, 91380 Chilly-Mazarin, France

In the last twenty years, two series of compounds have been discovered which exhibit marked diuretic and saluretic activity. These are (a) the phenoxyacetic acids, the most prominent member being ethacrynic acid (1,2, Figure 1) and (b) the sulfamoylbenzoic acids, the most potent being furosemide (3) and bumetanide (4,5). The latter compound differs from furosemide in several respects, the most obvious being that the 5-chloro substituent is replaced by phenoxy.

These very potent natriuretic agents are sufficiently effective to satisfy the physician for use in the treatment of hypertension and cardiac diseases; however, they possess unwanted side effects which include potassium depletion, a diabetogenic propensity (6,7,8,9) and hyperuricemia (10-23). To solve the problem of potassium depletion, a search for new diuretic agents led to the discovery of compounds which block the tubular sodium-potassium exchange either directly, i.e., triamterene (24) and amiloride (25), or by blocking the action of aldosterone, i.e., spironolactone.

In regard to diuretic-induced hyperuricemia, the discovery in 1967 of tienilic acid was a major contribution to diuretic therapy. This compound, /2,3-dichloro-4-(2-thienylcarbonyl)phenoxy/-acetic acid, is an aryloxyacetic acid analog of ethacrynic acid which exhibits diuretic and uricosuric activity in mice, rats and dogs (28), as well as in man (29,30,31). More recently, another aryloxyacetic acid, an indanone (32,33,34,35), has been reported to possess potent diuretic and uricosuric activity in chimpanzees and in man.

The purpose of the studies which we will describe was to evaluate the diuretic and uricosuric effects of tienilic acid in mice, rats and dogs and the antihypertensive properties in SH rats preliminary to clinical trials.

METHODS

Diuretic and Uricosuric Activity in Mice (36) - Initial screening

0-8412-0464-0/78/47-083-**056**$07.25/0

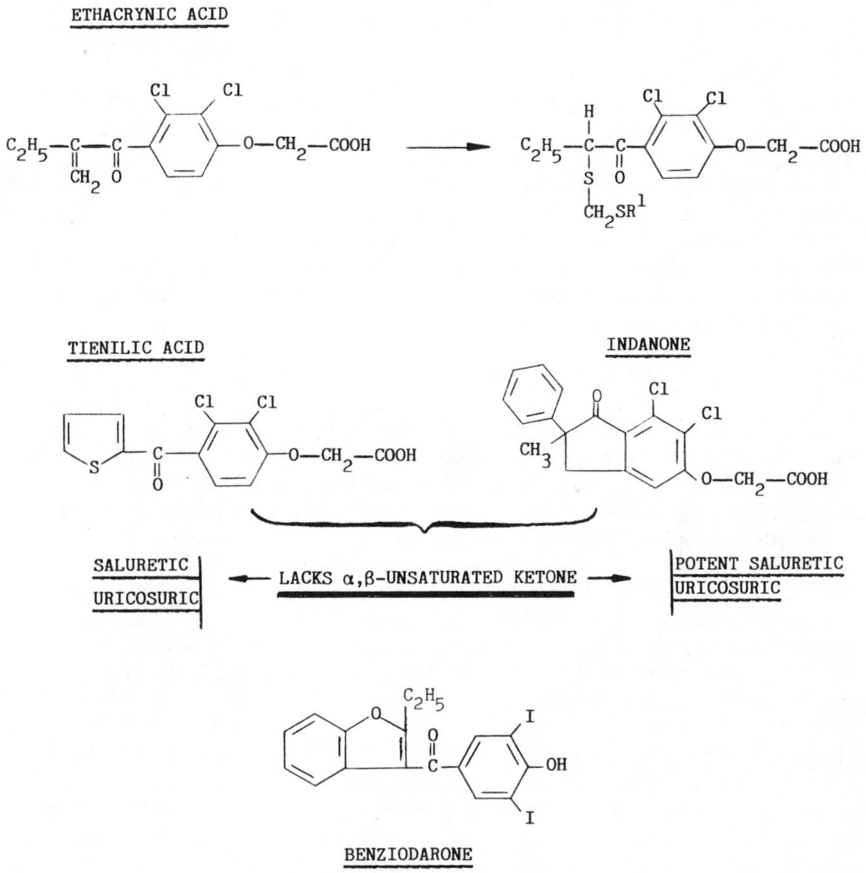

ETHACRYNIC ACID

TIENILIC ACID   INDANONE

| SALURETIC | ← LACKS α,β–UNSATURATED KETONE → | POTENT SALURETIC |
| URICOSURIC | | URICOSURIC |

BENZIODARONE

Figure 1. Compound structures

of diuretic agents were performed using groups of 6 male Swiss
mice, weighing 22 $\pm$ 1 g, randomly selected and distributed in
pairs into metabolism cages for 2 or 4 hours. Food and water were
withheld for 2 hours prior to the experiments, urine was collected
at 2 and 4 hours and the urine volumes and electrolytes measured.
All mice were administered 1 ml of 0.9% saline orally and either
simultaneously treated or not (control group) with diuretic
agents. Test compounds (tienilic acid, ethacrynic acid and
furosemide) were dissolved or suspended in the same 0.9% saline
and administered by gavage. Four groups received tienilic acid
orally at doses of 20, 50, 100 and 200 mg/kg and were compared to
furosemide at 20 mg/kg, ethacrynic acid at 20 mg/kg and
benziodarone (a potent non-diuretic uricosuric agent) at 100 mg/kg
by the same route. For the general screening of diuretic and
uricosuric drugs, such as tienilic acid and its congeners, the
compounds were administered at doses of 100 mg/kg orally in
comparison to furosemide or ethacrynic acid at 20 mg/kg.

Na^+ and K^+ analyses were determined using the flame photometer
(Eppendorf), chlorides by microanalysis (37) and uric acid by the
enzymatic spectrophotometric technique (38) or by a colorimetric
method (39). Statistical analysis was made by application of
Student's t test with simultaneous calculation of means (M) and
standard deviation of the mean (S/$\sqrt{n}$).

Tienilic Acid-Benziodarone and Furosemide-Benziodarone Relationships in Mice - Groups of 6 mice weighing 22 $\pm$ 1 g were administered simultaneously either 100 mg/kg or 200 mg/kg of tienilic
acid, or 200 mg/kg of benziodarone, or 20 mg/kg of furosemide or a
combination of the same doses of tienilic acid + benziodarone or
furosemide + benziodarone. After dosing, all animals were distributed by pairs into metabolism cages for 2 hours. Urine
samples were collected for the determination of electrolyte and
uric acid excretion using the same analytical methods as previously described. The statistical significance was based on a
comparison of tienilic acid + benziodarone or furosemide +
benziodarone versus tienilic acid alone, furosemide alone or
benziodarone alone (Student's t test).

Diuretic Activity in Rats - Groups of 3 animals weighing 400 $\pm$ 5
g, deprived of food and water overnight, were given 20 ml/kg of
water by intubation on the day preceding the experiment. After
dosing, the animals were placed in metabolism cages for the
collection of a 5 hour sample of urine. Diuretic drugs were
administered as in the previous experiment in a volume of 20 ml/kg
of 0.9% saline at the beginning of the experiment, while a control
group was administered only the saline solution. Statistical
significance refers to a comparison between treated and control
rats (Student's t test). Dose-response relationships are illustrated in Figure 5 using the regression line procedure.

Phenol-Red Retention Test in Rats (40,41) - Groups of 5 randomized
male rats, weighing 180 ± 20 g, were given the test compounds
orally 30 minutes before the intravenous injection of 75 mg/kg of
phenol-red as a 1.5% solution in 0.9% sodium chloride. Heparin-
ized blood samples were taken from the retro-orbital plexus at 15,
30, 45 and 60 minutes; color was developed by the addition of 0.05
ml of 0.1 M sodium hydroxide and read at 540 mμ on the spectro-
colorimeter (Eppendorf). Results were calculated as percentage of
variation in relation to the control value. Statistical significance was calculated by comparison with treated and control rats
(Student's t test).

Antihypertensive Activity in Spontaneous Hypertensive Rats
(Wistar-Okamoto Strain) - The studies were performed in Wistar
hypertensive male rats which were approximately 25 weeks old and
randomly placed in groups of six animals. The systolic blood
pressure was determined by the tail cuff technique (Physiograph
Narco System) before treatment and at 2, 5 and 24 hours after each
daily administration of the drug or the vehicle, in acute (1 day)
and in subacute experiments (8 days). In chronic studies, the
blood pressure was measured indirectly before and 1.5, 3.5, 6, 12
and 18 months after the beginning of the experiment. In the last
study, tienilic acid was mixed with the daily food at a level
calculated to provide an oral intake of 100 and 200 mg/kg.

In the acute oral experiments, the rats (N = 6) were given
100, 200 and 400 mg/kg of tienilic acid; in the subacute experiments, the daily oral dose was 200 mg/kg. Statistical analysis
was determined by Tukey's multiple comparisons procedure which
permits the statistical classification of means between themselves
or compared to control data. In Figure 17, statistical significance is illustrated by the addition of a broken line to the main
solid line. Each point represents a mean value, and the vertical
bars indicate the standard error of the mean.

In the chronic study, statistical significance was calculated
by Student's t paired test.

In all the experiments, the blood pressure was measured
indirectly in a control group of SH rats under the same conditions. In addition, in the chronic study, the treated SH rats were
compared to control Wistar normotensive rats.

Triglyceride-Lowering Effect in Obese Rats (Fatty Strain) -
Measurement of the triglyceride-lowering effect was carried out in
groups of 5 to 7 obese male rats (Fatty strain) and compared to
normal heterozygous rats as a first control group and to normal
Wistar rats as a second control group.

Obese rats were randomly distributed into two groups of 5 to
7 animals which were given either 200 mg/kg of tienilic acid as an
oral daily dose for 7 days or the vehicle alone. The other control
groups (heterozygous rats and normal Wistar rats) were given only
the fluid vehicle. Blood samples were taken at the end of the

experiment from the retro-orbital plexus in order to determine
plasma glucose, total lipids, cholesterol and triglyceride levels
after daily treatment with tienilic acid. Statistical significance was calculated in comparison with treated and control rats
(Student's t test).

Diuretic, Uricosuric and Clearance Studies in Anesthetized Beagle
Dogs under Hydropenic Conditions - The diuretic, uricosuric and
clearance studies were performed in beagle dogs weighing 10 to 13
kg which had been fasted overnight and then anesthetized by i.v.
injection of mebubarbital, 30 mg/kg. During the experiment, the
dogs were intravenously infused at a rate of 2 ml/minute with 0.6%
saline, 0.08% PAH, 0.4% creatinine and mebubarbital, 5 mg/kg/hour
using a constant rate infusion pump. After mesial laparotomy and
catheterization of the ureters, each study started with a control
period of two hours. Blood and urine samples were collected at 15
minute intervals. Then, the lysine salt of tienilic acid was
injected intravenously at 5, 10 and 20 mg/kg. A group of 4 to 6
beagle dogs was used for each dose and for the control (placebo)
evaluation. Sodium and potassium determinations were made using
the Eppendorf Flame Photometer, chloride by the colorimetric
micromethod (37) and urate by the enzymatic procedure (38). Other
measurements and calculations which were made are as follows: PAH
(42), creatinine (43), urea (44), pH, blood pressure, C_{osm} (osmolar clearance) after cryoscopic determination (using the freez-
ing point depression), $T^C H_2 O$ (free water reabsorption) and $T^C H_2 O =$
$C_{osm} - \dot{V}$ (ml/min). The $C_{osm} - T^C H_2 O$ relationship was studied
using $T^C H_2 O$ corrected for osmolar clearance and creatinine clearance as previously described (45): $\dfrac{T^C H_2 O / C_{osm}}{C_{creat.}}$. All the clear-

ance studies were determined using standard procedures. Statistical significance was calculated as previously described by the
application of Tukey's test (Section 5). Data are illustrated in
various figures as the mean values and the standard error of the
mean (vertical bars) or as percentage of control values.

RESULTS

Diuretic Activity in Mice - As shown in Figure 2, the oral administration of tienilic acid (20, 50, 100, 200 mg/kg p.o.) gave a
significant increase in urine volume and electrolyte excretion.
However, in comparison with furosemide or ethacrynic acid,
tienilic acid is about 1/5 to 1/10 as potent. Nevertheless,
contrary to other diuretic and natriuretic agents, tienilic acid
increases urate excretion.
        The uricosuric activity of tienilic acid in mice is dose-
related, as shown in Figure 3, in comparison with that of furosemide and ethacrynic acid in effective diuretic doses. In the same
experiment, benziodarone, which possesses significant uricosuric

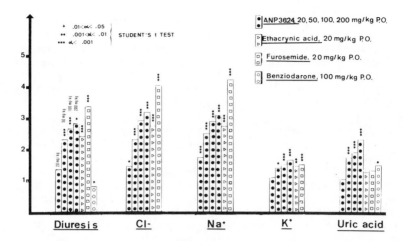

Figure 2.   ANP 3624 (tienilic acid–ticrynafen)—diuretic and uricosuric activity in the mouse

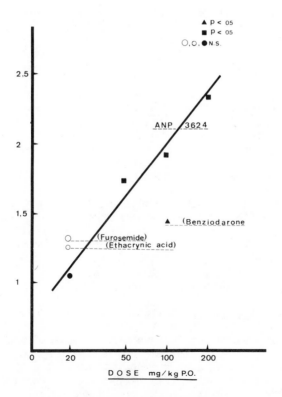

Figure 3.   ANP 3624 (tienilic acid–ticrynafen)—uricosuric activity in the mouse

properties in humans (46,67), has increased the urate excretion in
mice without greatly altering renal function. However, in the
benziodarone-tienilic acid interrelationship studies, it was
demonstrated that benziodarone inhibits the diuretic effect of
tienilic acid, but their uricosuric effects were synergistic
(Figure 4). Conversely, the benziodarone-furosemide combination
does not modify these parameters.

As seen in Table I, tienilic acid is the most active member
of this series, and only three compounds possess both diuretic and
uricosuric activities, i.e., ANP 3624 (tienilic acid), ANP 4316
(the 3-thienyl analogue of tienilic acid) and ANP 3860 (the
2-benzofuranyl analogue of tienilic acid). This latter compound,
which produced an increase in urate elimination along with a weak
natriuretic effect, possesses some of the structural features of
the 2,3-dichlorophenoxyacetic acids and some of those of
benziodarone, which is a benzofuran. From these studies, it is
obvious that tienilic acid has a specific effect on the urate
transport. This activity of the drug, initially observed in mice,
has been confirmed in rats and dogs.

Oral Diuretic Activity of Tienilic Acid in the Rat - As seen in
Figure 5 and according to many authors, ethacrynic acid was
ineffective at a dose as high as 300 mg/kg (Γ = .29 NS); tienilic
acid was weakly diuretic in doses up to 400 mg/kg $\sqrt{\Gamma}$ = .96 (P <
.05)7 and furosemide exhibited marked diuretic activity at a dose
of 50 mg/kg.

Uricosuric Activity of Tienilic Acid in the Rat as Measured by the
Phenol-Red Test - In view of the difficulties in administering
uric acid to small animals, the indirect method of Scarborough and
McKinney (41) for screening uricosuric agents in rats was used.
This indirect method does not measure the excretion of uric acid,
but rather the phenol-red retention induced by all uricosuric
substances.

In this test, as illustrated in Figure 6, tienilic acid and
benziodarone exhibited similar inhibition of phenol-red elimination, while furosemide and ethacrynic acid were ineffective. It
should be noted that in the same experiment probenecid and sulfinpyrazone reduced the phenol-red elimination and that acetyl-
salicylic acid strongly inhibited the activity of tienilic acid
and benziodarone (unpublished data).

Diuretic Activity in Anesthetized Beagle Dogs - Diuretic and
Natriuretic Activity - The acute effect of tienilic acid on urine
and electrolyte excretion in anesthetized beagle dogs is illustrated in Figures 7-11. Intravenous administration of 5, 10, 20
mg/kg of tienilic acid caused a statistically significant dose-
related excretion of urine (Figure 7) with an increase of renal
sodium (Figure 8), potassium (Figure 9) and chloride excretion
(Figure 10). At every dose, the sum of Na^+ and K^+ excretion was

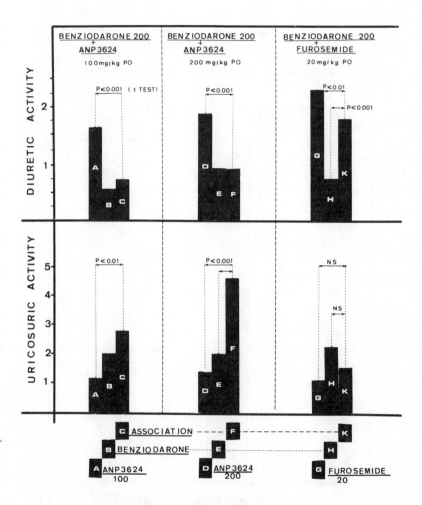

Figure 4. Antagonism benziodarone–ANP 3624 (diuresis) with synergistic increase of the uricosuric effect (mice N =6)

Table I

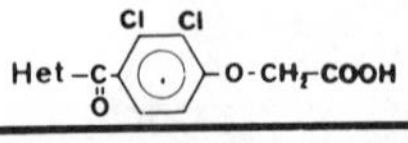

Het $-\overset{\overset{}{\underset{O}{||}}}{C}$ —⟨Cl Cl⟩— O-CH₂-COOH

A N P	HET.	DIURETIC ACTIVITY (MICE)				
		H_2O	$Na^•$	$K^•$	$\frac{Na^•}{K^•}$	urates
3624[**]	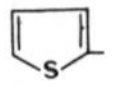 thiophene	2.7[*]	2.9[•]	1.5	1.9[•]	1.9[*]
3649	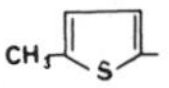 CH₃-thiophene	1.2	1.8	1.1	1.7	1
4357	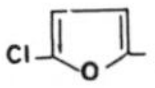 Cl-furan	.8	.7	.6	1.2	.9
3598[*]	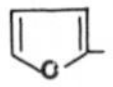 furan	1.8[*]	5.4[•]	1.5[•]	3.5[•]	1.1
4384	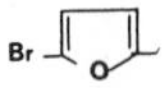 Br-furan	1.1	1.4	.8	1.7	1.1
4316[**]	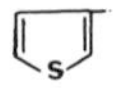 thiophene	2.7[*]	2.2[•]	1.9[•]	1.2	1.6[*]
4381[*]	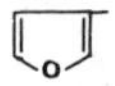 furan	1.6[*]	2	·1	1.8[•]	.9
4303	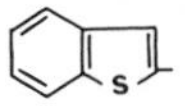 benzothiophene	1.2	1.2	.9	1.3	1.1
4294	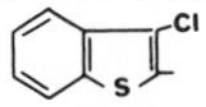 benzothiophene-Cl	1.3	1.3	1.2	1.1	1.3
3860[*]	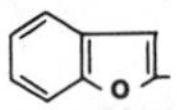 benzofuran	1.3	1.5[•]	1.7[•]	.9	1.6[*]
A[*]	ETACRYNIC ACID	2.4[*]	2.8[•]	1.5	1.9[•]	1·3
B[*]	FUROSEMIDE	3[*]	4.3[•]	1.5	2.8[•]	1.4

• , * , ★ , P< 0.05 STUDENT's t TEST

A , B 20 mg/kg PO

ANP 3624... 100 mg/kg PO

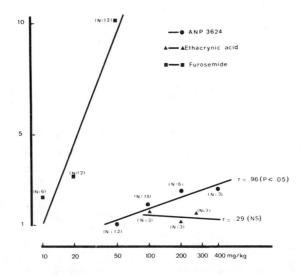

Figure 5. ANP 3624 (tienilic acid–ticrynafen)—diuretic activity in the normal rat

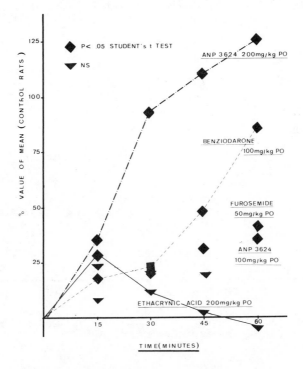

Figure 6. ANP 3624 (tienilic acid–ticrynafen)—retention of phenol red in the rat (N = 5)

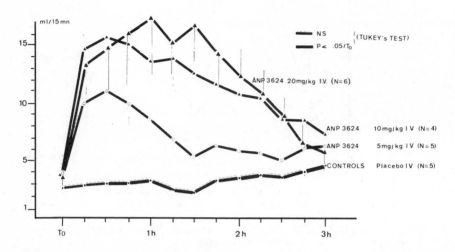

Figure 7.   ANP 3624 (tienilic acid–ticrynafen)—diuretic activity in the anesthetized beagle dog

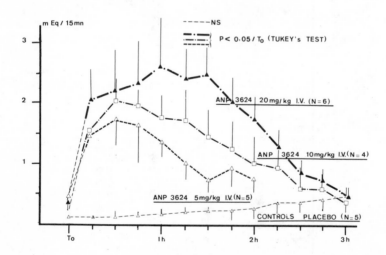

Figure 8.   ANP 3624 (tienilic acid–ticrynafen)—diuretic activity in the anesthetized beagle dog (Na⁺)

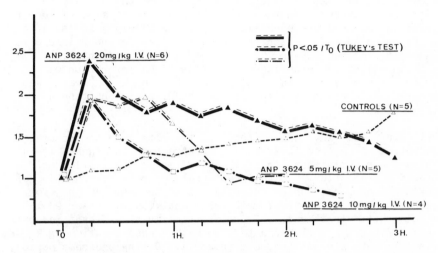

Figure 9. ANP 3624 (tienilic acid–ticrynafen)—diuretic activity in the anesthetized beagle dog (K^+)

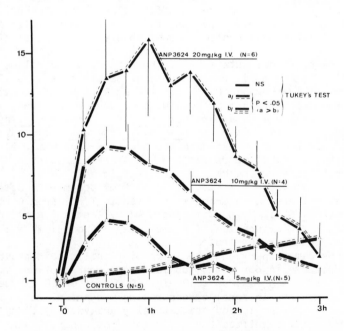

Figure 10. ANP 3624 (tienilic acid–ticrynafen)—diuretic activity in the anesthetized beagle dog (Cl^-)

about equal to that of chloride excretion and the urinary pH
remained unchanged. In these experiments, the total duration of
urine and electrolyte excretion was approximately 3 hours. After
intravenous administration, the maximal diuretic and natriuretic
response occurred within 30 minutes after drug injection.

In all of the experiments the rise of Na^+ excretion was
accompanied by a rise in K^+ excretion, but the Na^+/K^+ ratio was
generally increased as with each of the diuretic substances
(Figure 11).

Uricosuric Activity - The effects of tienilic acid on the urate
excretion in anesthetized beagle dogs are seen in Figures 12-14.
Intravenous administration of 10 and 20 mg/kg of tienilic acid
caused a statistically significant urate excretion. The time of
maximum increase in urine output is about the same as that for Na^+
excretion and the greatest uricosuric activity was observed 15
minutes after treatment, but a statistically significant response
lasted for 3 hours (Tukey's test). In this experiment, 5 mg/kg of
tienilic acid did not induce uricosuria. During the same period,
no statistically significant changes in creatinine clearance were
noted (Figures 13, 14).

Clearance Studies - As shown in Figures 13-15, tienilic acid at
i.v. doses of 5, 10 and 20 mg/kg affected renal clearances,
particularly osmolar clearance and free water reabsorption when
exogenous creatinine excretion showed no statistically significant
change.

In the hydropenic state, a slight rise of urine volume was
accompanied by marked increases in total solute clearance. This
effect, which is shown in Figure 15 (20 mg/kg i.v. of tienilic
acid), caused an increase in free water reabsorption. But, interestingly, when these data were corrected for osmolar clearance and
glomerular filtration rate, as previously suggested (45, 47-52),
tienilic acid proved to decrease the negative free water clearance
(Figure 16), i.e., it decreases free water reabsorption. In these
experiments, after 20 mg/kg i.v. of tienilic acid (N = 6), C_{osm}
increased from 0.60 ± 0.11 to 1.79 ± 0.26 ml per minute after 30
minutes when there was a progressive rise in $T^C H_2O$ from $0.40 \pm$
0.07 to 0.80 ± 0.11. Using data factored by C_{osm} and glomerular
filtration rate (Figure 16), $T^C H_2O$ decreased from 3.527 ± 1.028 to
1.410 ± 0.366 after 90 minutes.

In the same experiment, 10 mg/kg of tienilic acid provoked a
similar decrease in corrected tubular water reabsorption, i.e.,
dropping from 3.103 ± 1.258 to 0.918 ± 0.268 after 60 minutes.
These disturbances in renal concentrating mechanism, which are
summarized in Figure 16 and statistically analyzed by Tukey's
test, were still significantly different from control values 3
hours after the diuretic was given; thus, the administration of 5
mg/kg of tienilic acid led to a significant change in the free
water reabsorption.

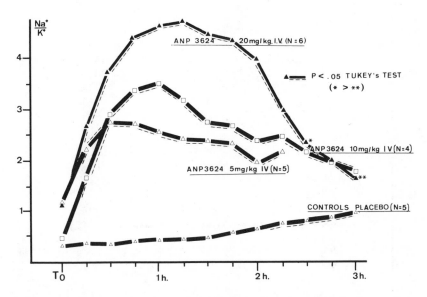

Figure 11.   ANP 3624 (tienilic acid–ticrynafen)—diuretic activity in the anesthetized beagle dog

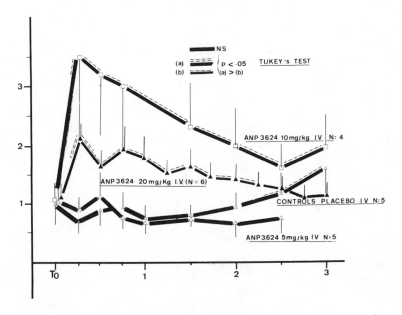

Figure 12.   ANP 3624 (tienilic acid–ticrynafen)—uricosuric activity in the anesthetized beagle dog

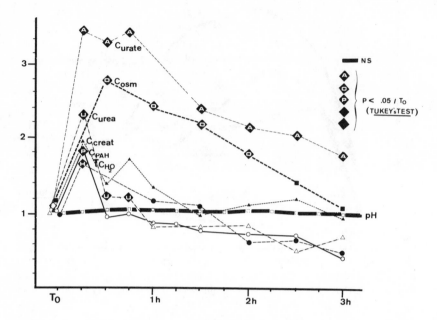

Figure 13. ANP 3624 (tienilic acid–ticrynafen)—10 mg/kg iv clearance studies
in the anesthetized beagle dog (N = 3–5)

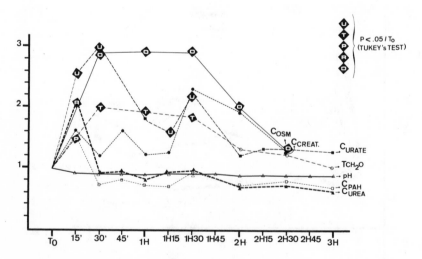

Figure 14. ANP 3624 (tienilic acid–ticrynafen)—20 mg/kg iv clearance studies
in the anesthetized beagle dog (N = 6)

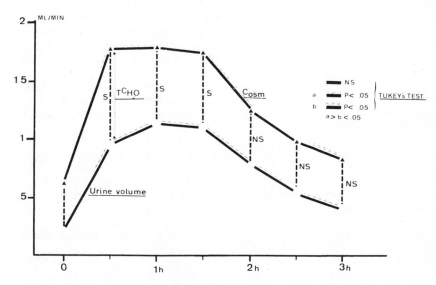

Figure 15.   ANP 3624 (tienilic acid–ticrynafen)—20 mg/kg iv (N = 6) = diuretic activity in the anesthetized beagle dog

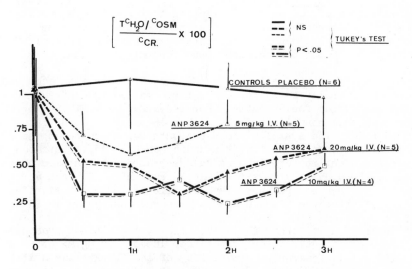

Figure 16.   ANP 3624 (tienilic acid–ticrynafen)—diuretic activity in the anesthetized beagle dog

During the same period, minor variations in PAH, creatinine and urea clearances were induced by 10 and 20 mg/kg of tienilic acid as demonstrated in Figures 13 and 14. Notably, the clearance of PAH increased from 71.38 ± 11.22 to 100.04 ± 29.99 and from 66.4 ± 13.03 to 121.27 ± 39.16 at 5 mg/kg and 20 mg/kg of tienilic acid, respectively. Under the same experimental conditions, the glomerular filtration rate slightly increased, i.e., the filtration fraction had a value between 0.35 and 0.50, or remained unchanged. The time required for the maximum change in PAH clearance was usually about 15-30 minutes after administration of tienilic acid.

Antihypertensive Activity of Tienilic Acid in the SH Rat - The combined diuretic, natriuretic and uricosuric properties of tienilic acid led to a study of its potential antihypertensive activity in SH rats using acute, subacute and chronic experiments in which the classic cuff technique was employed.

Acute Antihypertensive Activity (Figure 17) - The systolic blood pressure of SH rats was significantly (Tukey's test) decreased after 2, 5 and 24 hours following administration of 200 and 400 mg/kg of tienilic acid by the oral route. The placebo did not produce any change in blood pressure, and tienilic acid at 100 mg/kg significantly decreased the blood pressure only after 2 and 5 hours following administration of the drug.

Subacute Antihypertensive Activity - Figure 18 shows that daily administration of 200 mg/kg of tienilic acid for 5 days produced a sustained antihypertensive response in SH rats at each time interval during the experiment. Three days after withdrawal of the drug, the blood pressure returned to control values.

Chronic Antihypertensive Activity (Figure 19) - Tienilic acid was administered orally to SH rats in daily doses of 100 and 200 mg/kg (mixed with food) for 6 months. For 100 mg/kg, N = 27; 200 mg/kg, N = 29; control normal rats, (N.R.) N = 15 and control SH rats (SHR) N = 25. The systolic blood pressure was measured at the beginning and then after 1.5, 3.5 and 6 months. As illustrated in Figure 19, tienilic acid (200 mg/kg) decreased the systolic blood pressure ($P < 0.05$ - Tukey's test) in SH rats after 3.5 and 6 months. Neither control nor tienilic acid at 100 mg/kg significantly affected the blood pressure measured indirectly in SH rats.

Interestingly, after 20 months, the systolic blood pressure was not significantly altered by either 100 or 200 mg/kg of tienilic acid. However, the mortality of the SH rats was statistically less in the animals receiving 200 mg/kg of tienilic acid, T_{27}^{21} = 408; $0.01 < \alpha < 0.05$ /Wilcoxon's non-parametric procedure (53)/. The respective numbers of surviving animals were 12/15 (normotensive Wistar rats), 4/21 (control SH rats), 16/27

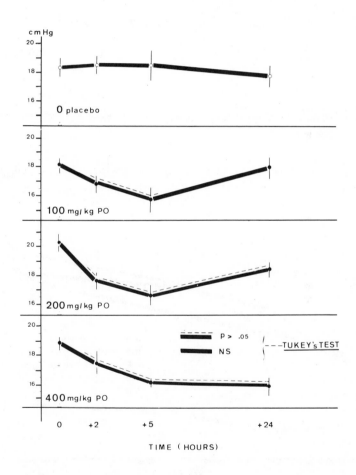

Figure 17. ANP 3624 (tienilic acid–ticrynafen)—acute antihypertensive activity in the SH rat (N = 6)

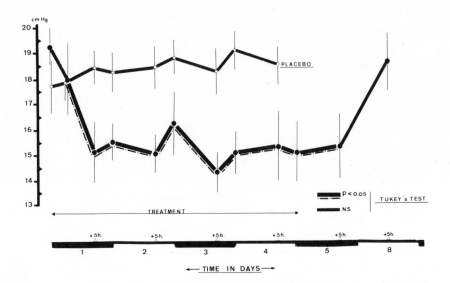

Figure 18.   ANP 3624 (tienilic acid–ticrynafen)—200 mg/kg/day po—antihypertensive activity in the SH rat (N = 6)

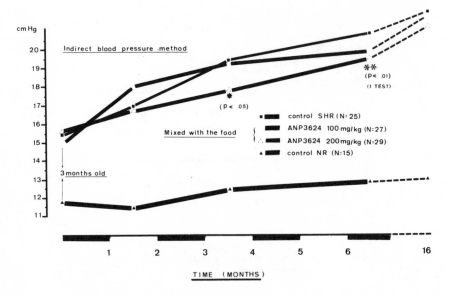

Figure 19.   ANP 3624 (tienilic acid–ticrynafen)—antihypertensive activity.   Chronic
study in the SH rat (♂).

(tienilic acid at 200 mg/kg) and 5/26 (tienilic acid at 100 mg/kg).

Blood Triglyceride-Lowering Effect in the Obese Rats (Fatty Strain) - In previous experiments, Maass (74) found that tienilic acid decreases the blood levels of triglycerides in normal rats. A similar activity has been found again in obese rats (Fatty Strain), but not in normal rats (Figure 20). However, total lipids, blood cholesterol and glucose levels remained unchanged in both animal models.

DISCUSSION

This paper describes the diuretic, natriuretic and uricosuric studies carried out over a period of years (28) in a variety of animals, including mice, rats and dogs. Recent pharmacological and clinical reports have confirmed the original observations (54-63) of Masbernard (29) who first reported the human pharmacological studies on this drug.

As shown in mice, rats and anesthetized beagle dogs, tienilic acid (ANP 3624), in contrast to furosemide, ethacrynic acid, the indanone and bumetanide, is a mild saluretic-diuretic agent at relatively high doses. But, in all the species studied in these experiments, tienilic acid exhibited the potent uricosuric activity required to decrease hyperuricemia, which is a cardiovascular risk factor.

In mice, the diuretic, uricosuric and natriuretic activities of tienilic acid were found to be dose-dependent (Figure 3); in normal rats, tienilic acid, in contradistinction to ethacrynic acid, provoked a dose-related diuretic and natriuretic response. In the same animal, this diuretic agent decreased phenol-red elimination, which has been regarded as an indirect measurement of a competitive antagonist of urate excretion in dogs, occurring mainly in the proximal tubule (64,65,66). This potential uricosuric activity as measured in the rat by antagonism of phenol-red elimination has been demonstrated by Lemieux (62) in a recent report which reveals that tienilic acid provoked a uricosuric effect in man, mouse, rat and dog (all species where urate reabsorption predominates). Indeed, in anesthetized beagle dogs, under hydropenic conditions, tienilic acid exhibits both diuretic and uricosuric properties over a wide dose range.

The diuretic activity was distinguished by a marked increase in water and Na^+ elimination with significant K^+ and Cl^- excretion. But, it was of interest to note that clearance studies showed a frank rise in both urate and osmolar clearances. This renders tienilic acid unique among the known diuretic agents, with the exception of another aryloxyacetic acid derivative, i.e., the indanone which also exhibited potent diuretic and uricosuric activities in chimpanzees and human subjects (32,33,34,35). As demonstrated in previous reports by other authors (54,60),

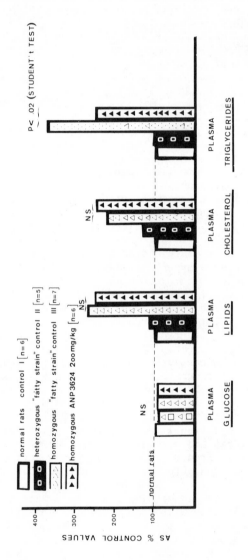

Figure 20. ANP 3624 (tienilic acid–ticrynafen)—200 mg/kg daily po (5 days)—study on the blood triglycerides lowering effect in the obese rat (fatty strain)

tienilic acid affects reabsorption and secretion of urate in dogs mainly in the proximal tubule. Other studies concerning the site of action of several non-diuretic uricosuric agents suggested the same conclusions (65,66,67,68). Inhibition of phenol-red excretion in rats by uricosuric agents and by diuretic-uricosuric substances indicates that they specifically depress urate reabsorption at the proximal site (64,65,66).

On the other hand, as summarized in Figure 15, tienilic acid exhibited a greater increase in osmolar clearance than in water excretion. Consequently, the calculated $T^C H_2O$ was significantly raised, as reported by Stote et al (54) and to a lesser degree by Maass et al (59). In conjunction with the previous data on $^C H_2O$, tienilic acid produced alterations in the cortical diluting segment of the distal nephron, unlike the other loop diuretics. However, when the reabsorption of solute free-water ($T^C H_2O$) was factored by osmolar clearance ($^C osm$) and glomerular filtration rate ($^C creat$) as previously reported (45, 47-52), free water reabsorption was surprisingly decreased by the administration of tienilic acid (Figures 15 and 16). A similar reversal was obtained when $T^C H_2O$ was corrected for osmolar clearance alone, attenuating the possible prominent part played by the creatinine clearance rate on the genesis of this phenomenon.

In the first absolute calculation of $T^C H_2O$ as it obtained from $^C osm$, the action of tienilic acid was qualitatively similar to that of chlorothiazide. Using the corrected $T^C H_2O$, the tienilic acid results were approximately similar to those of ethacrynic acid and furosemide, while they were opposite to those of the thiazides. Considering these results in the light of the properties of tienilic acid in a hydrated state, these corrected calculations of $T^C H_2O$ do not exclude the possibility that tienilic acid could alter an additional site in the renal tubule. In an attempt to support this assumption, it is interesting to note that the calculation of both corrected $^C H_2O$ and $T^C H_2O$ from data reported in papers from several investigators, no change in the normal increase of hydrochlorothiazide activity on solute-free water reabsorption (69) was seen. On the other hand, the corrected calculations reversed the rather mild effect of tienilic acid on $T^C H_2O$ similar to that seen in the present study (54) and restored the $^C H_2O$ to the expected values for furosemide (70,71) and chlormerodrine (72) which, displayed paradoxically, altered absolute $^C H_2O$ values. More exactly, the corrected calculations of $^C H_2O$ and $T^C H_2O$ have normalized the paradoxical effects observed for furosemide or chlormerodrine, while the same corrections reversed the significance of the effects of tienilic acid in regard to solute-free water reabsorption. For example, in the experiment of Stote et al (54), tienilic acid very moderately increased the $T^C H_2O$ before the correction, and significantly decreased the $T^C H_2O$ value using the same calculation, while $^C H_2O$ in water diuresis was not modified when an analogous calculation was made with respect to urinary flow and inulin clearance. In the same way, in the report

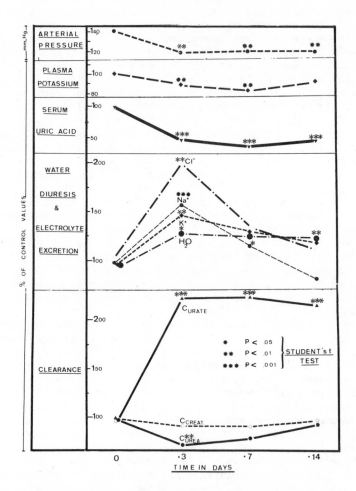

Figure 21. Tienilic acid (250–750 mg daily)—antihypertensive
and uricosuric effect in essential hypertensive patients (N = 12)
(64)

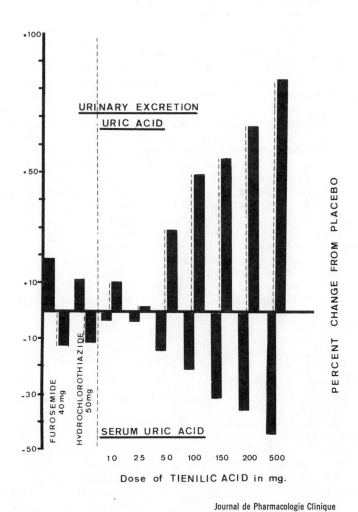

Journal de Pharmacologie Clinique

Figure 22. Tienilic acid—effect on uric acid in man—serum values and urinary excretion (54)

of Suki et al (70), using $_c$furosemide at 2 mg/kg i.v. paradoxically
increased the calculated ^{c}H$_2$O in dogs but markedly decreased the
experimental value. However, in the report of Azer et al (71),
which describes the proximal tubular rejection of sodium by
furosemide, chlormerodrine, 8 mg/kg, did not change the T^{c}H$_2$O
because of paradoxical data generated by his three experiments;
but after correction, chlormerodrine depressed significantly
solute-free water reabsorption in comparison to the control value.

In conclusion, it is suggested that these data are consistent
with the idea that under some conditions of urinary excretion,
tienilic acid possesses an additional site of action. On the
other hand, it is of interest to observe that there is a good
parallelism between the animal data and the clinical studies, as
shown in Figures 21 and 22, which confirm the diuretic, uricosuric
and antihypertensive properties of tienilic acid in man. It
should be noted that the hypouricemia seen in man has not been
observed in small rodents and dogs.

Finally, the combined diuretic, uricosuric, antihypertensive
and triglyceride-lowering properties of tienilic acid observed in
rats suggest that the control of these factors as risks in cardiac
diseases may explain the increase of survival time of SH rats
after chronic administration of tienilic acid.

Literature Cited

1. Schultz, E. M., Cragoe, E. J., Jr., Bicking, J. B., Bolhofer, W. A. and Sprague, J. M., J. Med. Pharm. Chem. (1962), 5, 660.
2. Baer, J. E., Michaelson, J. K., McKinstry, D. N. and Beyer, K. H., Proc. Soc. Exp. Biol. Med. (1964), 115, 87-90.
3. Kleinfelder, H., Ger. Med. (1963), 8, 459.
4. Feit, P. W., J. Med. Chem. (1971), 14, 432.
5. Feit, P. W. and Tvaermose Nielsen, O. B., J. Med. Chem. (1972), 15, 79.
6. Wilkins, R. W., Ann. Int. Med. (1959), 50, 1.
7. Goldner, M. G. H., Zarowitz, H., Akgun, S., N. Engl. J. Med. (1960), 262, 403.
8. Shapiro, A. P., Benedek, T. G., Small, J. L., N. Engl. J. Med. (1960), 265, 1028.
9. Lyon, A. F., DeGraff, A. C., Am. Heart J. (1964), 68, 710.
10. Hartmann, F. and Heimsoth, V., "Antihypertensive Therapy", 436-447. Proceedings edited by F. Gross, Springer-Verlag, 1966.
11. DeMartini, F. E., Arthritis and Rheum. (1965), 8, 823-829.
12. Carmon, P. J., Heinemann, H. O., Stason, W. B., Laragh, J. H., Circulation (1965), 31, 5.
13. Stason, W. B., Carmon, P. J., Heinemann, H. O. and Laragh, J. H., Circulation (1966), 34, 190-200.
14. Humphreys, M. B., Br. Med. J. (1966), 1, 1024-1025.
15. McKenzie, F. C., Fairley, K. F., Baird, C. W., Med. J. Aus. (1966), 879-886.
16. Hutcheon, D. E., Mehta, D., Romano, A., Arch. Int. Med. Exp. (1965), 115, 542-546.
17. Bryant, J. M., Fan Yu, T., Berger, L., Schwartz, N.,

Torosdag, S., Fletcher, L., Fertig, H., Schwartz, S., Quan, F. B. F., Am. J. Med. (1962), 33, 408.

18. Kim, K. E., Onesti, G., Mayer, J. H., Schwartz, C., Am. J. Cardiol. (1971), 27, 407.

19. Olesen, K. H., Sigurd, B., Steiness, E., Leth, A., Acta Med. Scand. (1973), 193, 119-131.

20. Steele, T. H., Rheumatic Diseases (1977), 3, 37-50.

21. Bourke, E., Asbury, M. J. A., O'Sullivan, S. and Gatenby, P. B. B., Eur. J. Pharmacol. (1973), 23, 283-289.

22. Davies, D. L., Lant, A. F., Millard, N. R., Smith, A. J., Ward, J. W. and Wilson, G. M., Clin. Pharmacol. Ther. (1973), 15, 141-155.

23. Hutcheon, D. E., Pocelinke, R. and Duchin, K. L., "New Antihypertensive Drugs", 323-336, A. Scriabine and C. S. Sweet. Spectrum Publications, Inc., New York, 1976.

24. Wiebelhaus, V. D., Weinstock, J., Brennan, F. T., Sosnowski, G. and Larsen, T. J., Fed. Proc. (1961), 20, 409.

25. Baer, J. E., Jones, C. B., Spitzer, S. A. and Russo, H. F., J. Pharmacol. Exp. Ther. (1967), 157, 472-485.

26. French Patent 2068403 (1973).

27. Godfroid, J. J. and Thuillier, J. E., U.S. Patent 3,758,506 (1973).

28. Thuillier, G. Laforest, J., Cariou, B. Bessin, P., Bonnet, J. and Thuillier, J., Eur. J. Med. Chem. Chim. Ther. (1974), 9, 625-633.

29. Masbernard, A. and Guidicelli, C., Lyon Med. (1974), 232, 165-174.

30. Stote, R. M., Cherrill, D. A., Erb, B. B. and Alexander, F., Clin. Res. (1974), 22, 721A.

31. Stote, R. M., Cherrill, D. A., Maass, A. R., Erb, B. B., Familiar, R. G. and Alexander, F., Abs. 6th Int. Cong. Neph., Florence, Italy, (1975) 827.

32. Cragoe, E. J., Jr., Schultz, E. M., Schneeberg, J. D., Stokker, G. E., Woltersdorf, O. W., Fanelli, G. M. and Watson, L. S., J. Med. Chem. (1974), 18, 225-228.

33. Woltersdorf, O. W., Schneeberg, J. D., Cragoe, E. J., Jr., Schultz, E. M., Stokker, G. E., Watson, L. S. and Fanelli, G. M., Abs. 169th Am. Chem. Soc. Nat. Mtg., Philadelphia, Pa., (1975) No. 49.

34. Woltersdorf, O. W., Cragoe, E. J., Jr., Watson, L. S. and Fanelli, G. M., Abs. 169th Am. Chem. Soc. Nat. Mtg., Philadelphia, Pa., (1975) No. 48.

35. Watson, L. S., Fanelli, G. M., Russo, H. F., Sweet, C. S., Ludden, C. T., Scriabine, A., "New Antihypertensive Drugs", 307-321, A. Scriabine and C. S. Sweet, Spectrum Publications, Inc., New York, 1976.

36. Bessin, P., Tetu, O. and Selim, M., Chim. Ther. (1969), 4 (3), 220.

37. Schales, O. and Schales, S., J. Biol. Chem. (1941), 140, 879.

38. Kageyama, N., Clin. Chim. Acta. (1971), 31 (2), 421.

39. Caraway, W. T., Am. J. Clin. Pathol. (1955), 25, 840. 40.
Kreppel, E., Med. Exp. (1959), 1, 285. 41. Scarborough, H. C. and
McKinney, G. R., J. Med. Pharm. Chem. (1962), 5, 175. 42.
Hamburger, J., Ryckewaert, A., Duysent, M. and Argant, N., Ann.
Biol. Clin. (Paris) (1948), 6, 358. 43. Popper, H., Mandel, E.
and Mayer, H., Biochem. Z. (1937), 291, 354.
44. Fawcett, J. K. and Scott, J. E., J. Clin. Pathol. (1960), 13,
156.
45. Carriere, S. and Dandavino, R., Clin. Pharmacol. and Ther.
(1976), 20 (4), 424-438.
46. Nivet, M., Marcovici, J. and Laruelle, F., Bull. Mem. Soc.
Med. Hop. Paris (1965), 116, 1187.
47. Goldberg, M., McCurdy, D. K., Foltz, E. L. and Bluemle, L.
W., J. Clin. Invest. (1964), 43, 201-216.
48. Suki, W., Rector, F. C., Jr. and Seldin, D. W., J. Clin.
Invest. (1965), 44, 1458-1469.
49. Stein, J. H., Wilson, C. B. and Kirkendall, W. M., J. Lab.
Clin. Med. (1968), 71, 654-665.
50. Puschett, J. B. and Goldberg, M., J. Lab. Clin. Med. (1968),
71, 666-677.
51. Martinez-Maldonado, M., Suki, W. N. and Schenker, S., Am. J.
Physiol. (1969), 216, 1376-1391.
52. Bourke, E., Asbury, M. J. A., O'Sullivan, S. and Gatenby, P.
B. B., Eur. J. Pharmacol. (1973), 23, 283-289.
53. Wilcoxon, F. and Wilcox, R. A., "Some Rapid Approximate
Statistical Procedures", American Cyanamid Company, Pearl River,
New York, 1964.
54. Stote, M., Maass, A. R., Cherrill, D. A., Beg, M. M. A. and
Alexander, F., J. Pharmacol. Clin. (1976), Special Issue, 19-27.
55. Masbernard, A., Giudicelli, C. P. and Kamaludin, T., J.
Pharmacol. Clin. (1976), Special Issue, 13-18.
56. Reese, O. G. and Steele, T. H., Am. J. Med. (1976), 60,
973-979.
57. Jain, A. K., Ryan, J. R. and McMahon, F. G., Clin. Res.
(1876), 24,1.
58. Steele, T. H., Prasad, D. R. and Reese, O. G., Clin.
Pharmacol. Ther. (1976), 19, 116.
59. Maass, A. R., Erickson, R., Snow, I., Brennan, F., Weedon, R.
and Hutchings, G., Physiologist (1976), 19, 280.
60. Stote, R., Goldberg, M. and Agus, Z. S., Clin. Res. (1976),
24, 405A.
61. Gillies, A., Morgan, G. and Morgan, T., Aust. N. Z. J. Med.
(1977), 7, 443-444.
62. Nemati, M. Kyle, M. C. and Freis, E. D., J. Am. Med. Assoc.
(1977), 237, 652-657.
63. Lemieux, G., Kiss, A., Vinay, P. and Gougoux, A., Kidney Int.
(1977), 12, 104-114.
64. Springinsfeld, M., Durel, J., Rieffel, R., and Jahn, H., J.
Pharmacol. Clin. (1976), Special Issue, 35-45.
65. Marshall, E. K., Am. J. Physiol. (1931), 99, 77.

66. Zins, G. R. and Weiner, I. M., Am. J. Physiol. (1968), 215, 411-422. 67. Weiner, I. M. and Fanelli, G. M., "Recent Advances in Physiology and Pharmacology", 53-68, Wessin, L. G. and Fanelli, G. M., Eds., University Park Press, 1974. 68. Lemieux, G., Gougoux, A., Vinay, P. and Michaud, G., Am. J. Physiol. (1973), 224, 1431-1439.
69. Lemieux, G., Vinay, P., Gougoux, A. and Michaud, G., Am. J. Physiol. (1973), 224, 1440-1449.
70. Early, L. E., Kahn, M. and Orloff, J., J. Clin. Invest. (1961), 40, 857-866.
71. Suki, W. N., Rector, F. C. and Seldin, D. W., J. Clin. Invest. 1965), 44, 1458-1469.
72. Azer, M. and Kirkendal, W. M., J. Pharmacol. Exp. Ther. (1973), 185, 235-244.
73. Puschett, J. B. and Goldberg, M., J. Lab. Clin. Med. (1968), 71, 666-677..
74. Maass, A. R., private communication.

RECEIVED August 21, 1978.

6

Ticrynafen: An Antihypertensive, Diuretic, Uricosuric Agent

A. R. MAASS, I. B. SNOW, and R. ERICKSON

Smith Kline and French Laboratories, 1500 Spring Garden St., Philadelphia, PA 19101

R. M. STOTE

Presbyterian-University of Pennsylvania Medical Center, Philadelphia, PA 19104

It is apparent that from a perusal of the articles in this publication that it is no longer sufficient to synthesize chemical structures which are modifications of existing diuretics in anticipation of obtaining a compound with similar diuretic activity. Examples of diuretics with markedly different chemical structures such as: mersalyl (1), ethacrynic acid (2), furosemide (3) and bumetanide (4), all of which act at the same site in the renal tubule have been known for some time. However, we also now know of two dichlorophenoxyacetic acid diuretics which act at different sites within the kidney tubule.

Ticrynafen is /2,3-dichloro-4-(2-thienylcarbonyl)phenoxy/-acetic acid. It was registered with the World Health Organization as tienilic acid; the USAN approved name, however, is ticrynafen. On the basis of its dichlorophenoxyacetic acid structure, it appears to be related to ethacrynic acid, /2,3-dichloro-4-(2-methylenebutyryl)phenoxy/acetic acid, but is chemically and pharmacologically quite different. For example, ethacrynic acid reacts avidly in vitro with the sulfhydryl amino acid, cysteine, while ticrynafen is quite inert. Since Burg (5) and others (6) have shown that it is the ethacrynic acid-cysteine adduct which is the active diuretic (at least in vitro), we were led to the conclusion that the two compounds would differ pharmacologically just as they differed chemically.

A pharmacologic difference was strongly suggested by our early observations on the effect of ticrynafen on diuretic and natriuretic activity in the mongrel dog. Ticrynafen, administered to the hydrated dog at doses of 12.5, 25 and 50 mg/kg orally, was compared, in an incomplete latin block design, with ethacrynic acid at oral doses of 3.1, 6.25 and 12.5 mg/kg. Urine was collected from these dogs for 5 hours and then for an additional 19 hours, for a total of 24 hours. Compared for diuretic and natriuretic effectiveness at 5 hours, ticrynafen was 1/26th and 1/23rd as active, respectively, as ethacrynic acid. However, after 24 hours collection, ticrynafen was 1/11th as active a diuretic and 1/14th as active a natriuretic agent as ethacrynic

0-8412-0464-0/78/47-083-**084**$05.00/0

acid. These data demonstrated that not only did the two compounds differ in duration of action, with ticrynafen being an
effective diuretic and natriuretic over a longer time span than
ethacrynic acid, but also suggested that the natriuretic potency
of ticrynafen differed from ethacrynic acid.

Since the response to a diuretic is principally determined
by the locus in the nephron where the drug exerts its inhibitory
effect on sodium reabsorption (7), we attempted to establish the
site of renal action of ticrynafen. There are four major sites
of diuretic activity in the renal tubule: a proximal site; two
sites, medullary and cortical, in the thick ascending limb of the
loop of Henle; and a far distal so-called sodium-potassium
exchange site. At one time or another, practically every site in
the tubule has been claimed as the active site for every diuretic
(8). But, in recent years, it has been accepted that the pattern
of electrolyte excretion, along with the determination of osmolal
clearance in hydrated and dehydrated animals or man, will charac-
terize the site of diuretic activity of a compound (7).

Adult female mongrel dogs were hydrated by giving an oral
water load of 500 ml tap water thirty minutes prior to initiation
of standard renal clearance procedure. Dogs were infused intravenously at 3 ml/minute throughout the course of the experiment
with a 4% mannitol-phosphate buffer solution, pH 7.4 (9). Glomerular filtration rate was determined by the clearance of
creatinine and effective renal plasma flow by the clearance of
p-aminohippurate. Ticrynafen, administered intravenously to four
hydrated mongrel dogs, caused a moderate natriuresis, kaliuresis
and chloruresis with only a nominal increase in urine volume.
The small change in urine flow rate above control (Table I)
suggested that ticrynafen had little or no proximal activity. In
this, ticrynafen differed from hydrochlorothiazide, furosemide
and acetazolamide. All of these compounds increased sodium
excretion which resulted in a positive osmolal clearance above
controls (n = 6). However, only acetazolamide caused a positive
free water clearance. These data suggested that ticrynafen was
active in the thick ascending limb of the loop of Henle.

TABLE I

DIURETIC EFFECTIVENESS IN HYDRATED DOGS

Drug	Diuresis* ml/min	Sodium* FE %	C_{osm}* ml/min	C_{H_2O}* ml/min
Acetazolamide	3.2	3.3	+ 1.4	+ 1.8
Furosemide	10.0	15.6	+14.2	− 4.2
Hydrochlorothiazide	1.8	5.3	+ 4.4	− 2.5
Ticrynafen (n = 4)	0.2	6.3	+ 3.8	− 3.6

* change from control

Adult, female mongrel dogs and dalmation coach hounds were fasted overnight. Using a constant rate infusion pump, the dogs were infused intravenously at 0.5 ml/minute throughout the course of the experiment with a 4% mannitol-phosphate buffer pH 7.4. The same standard renal clearance procedures were followed except that urine collection intervals were 20 minutes rather than the 10 minute collection periods used in the hydrated dogs. In the hydropenic dogs; however, ticrynafen is readily distinguished from furosemide by its lack of a significant affect upon T^cH_2O, the solute free water of reabsorption. Ticrynafen, administered intravenously at 15 mg/kg to eight hydropenic dogs increased urine flow rate above that of the controls (Table II) in the protocol. Again, the natriuretic effectiveness of ticrynafen was equivalent to that of hydrochlorothiazide, and again it increased osmolal clearance. However, the modest change on free water of reabsorption (T^cH_2O) strongly suggested a site of activity in the cortical diluting segment of the distal tubule.

TABLE II

DIURETIC EFFECTIVENESS IN HYDROPENIC DOGS

Drug	Diuresis ml/min	Sodium FE %	C_{osm} ml/min	T^cH_2O ml/min
Acetazolamide	1.8	3.4	+ 2.5	+ 0.7
Furosemide	4.0	5.9	+ 3.6	- 0.4
Hydrochlorothiazide	0.9	3.0	+ 1.7	+ 0.8
Ticrynafen (n = 8)	1.5	3.2	+ 1.6	+ 0.1

Similar data have been obtained in the hydrated and dehydrated normal male volunteer (10). Ticrynafen at 500 or 1000 mg had no effect upon urine flow rate in the hydrated volunteers (Table III), suggesting a lack of proximal activity. Ticrynafen, given orally to hydrated subjects, increased sodium excretion and osmolal clearance but decreased free water clearance.

TABLE III

DIURETIC EFFECTIVENESS IN HYDRATED NORMAL VOLUNTEERS

Dose	Diuresis ml/min	Sodium FE %	C_{osm} ml/min	C_{H_2O} ml/min
Control	16.0	1.3	3.4	12.8
500 mg (n = 3)	16.1	4.3	7.1	8.9
Control	15.0	1.0	3.3	11.8
1000 mg (n = 2)	14.7	5.7	7.7	6.9

In hydropenic volunteers, ticrynafen, at 500 or 1000 mg orally, also increased sodium excretion and osmolal clearance. Unlike free water clearance however, tubular reabsorption of solute free water rose and was either equal to or exceeded that of the controls (Table IV). This observation, along with the observation in both hydrated and hydropenic normal volunteers, that only 4 to 6% of the filtered sodium load was excreted, clearly place the site of diuretic activity of ticrynafen in the cortical diluting segment of the distal tubule (10).

TABLE IV

DIURETIC EFFECTIVENESS IN HYDROPENIC NORMAL VOLUNTEERS

Dose	Diuresis ml/min	Sodium FE %	C_{osm} ml/min	$T^{C}H_2O$ ml/min
Control	0.9	0.9	3.0	2.1
500 mg (n = 3)	3.3	4.6	6.4	3.1
Control	0.9	1.1	3.1	2.2
1000 mg (n = 2)	4.7	6.1	6.9	2.2

The congruence of results of activity of ticrynafen in hydrated and hydropenic man and dog upon free water clearance and the solute free water of reabsorption delineate its site of action (Table V). Proximal, loop and distal diuretics administered to hydrated dogs increased sodium excretion and osmolal clearance. Based on the physiologic principles outlined by Goldberg et al. (11), free water clearance (C_{H_2O}) was increased only by acetazolamide, a proximally active diuretic (12) and was decreased by loop and distally acting diuretics. But in hydropenic animals, the distally active compounds, hydrochlorothiazide and ticrynafen caused a slight increase or no change in $T^{C}H_2O$, clearly a different response than that obtained with furosemide (13), a "loop-agent".

TABLE V

SUMMARY OF THE EFFECTS OF DIURETICS UPON
RENAL CONCENTRATING AND DILUTING MECHANISMS

| | Experimental Procedure | |
Site of Action	Hydropenic $T^{C}H_2O$	Hydrated C_{H_2O}
Proximal Tubule Acetazolamide	↑	↑
Loop of Henle Furosemide	↓	↓
Distal Tubule Ticrynafen	±	↓

To determine the pattern of electrolyte excretion in the
dog, ticrynafen was administered intravenously, in single acute
doses, to the phosphate-mannitol infused dog. At intravenous
doses of 0.05 to 15 mg/kg, the compound enhanced urine volume
and caused excretion of sodium, potassium and chloride. The
maximum natriuretic response occurred promptly within the first
10 minutes after completion of the injection, and as the dose
was increased there was a greater duration of natriuresis
(Table VI).

TABLE VI

ELECTROLYTE EXCRETION FOLLOWING ADMINISTRATION OF
TICRYNAFEN TO THE PHOSPHATE-MANNITOL INFUSED DOG

I. V. Dose mg/kg	No of Observations	Maximal FE Na %	Total Cumulative Excretion mEq During First Hour		
			Na	K	Cl
Placebo	10	2.09	5.29	1.49	2.64
0.05	3	2.93	9.39	1.36	6.33
0.5	6	3.91	7.02	1.13	4.00
2.5	1	7.40	12.96	2.80	11.61
5.0	4	10.05	19.31	2.09	15.46
15.0	3	11.60	33.85	4.58	31.80

When compared statistically with placebo, ticrynafen caused
a significant natriuretic response at 0.5 mg/kg I.V. which
increased in a linear fashion with dose, reaching a maximum
effect with excretion of about 12% of the filtered sodium load
at 15 mg/kg. The excretion of chloride parallels that of sodium
but is somewhat reduced due to the presence of phosphate in the
infusion-medium, suggesting that ticrynafen is a saluretic

agent. A significant increase in potassium excretion occurred at a dose of 2.5 mg/kg, five times the minimum effective natriuretic dose. This observation makes it unlikely that ticrynafen has an inhibitory affect upon the sodium/potassium exchange site.

During maximal natriuresis in man, following administration of 500 mg ticrynafen, average sodium excretion increased 463 µEq/min., while potassium excretion increased only 16 µEq/min. Clearance ratio of calcium to inulin increased by approximately 1% and clearance ratio of magnesium 2.6%. Bicarbonate and phosphorus excretions were not significantly changed, and urinary pH consistently decreased. The acute administration of ticrynafen did not result in any significant change in GFR as determined by inulin clearance. This electrolyte pattern again supports a conclusion of a lack of activity of ticrynafen in the proximal tubule, while the similarity of electrolyte response to "thiazide-like" diuretics is consistent with an action in the cortical diluting segment of the distal tubule.

As a result of these observations, we have concluded that hydrochlorothiazide and ticrynafen, two compounds with markedly differing chemical structure, produce a similar pattern of electrolyte response due to their activity at the same site in the kidney tubule.

While diuretics of markedly differing chemical structure have not been recognized previously to be active at a <u>cortical</u> diluting site, compounds of widely differing structure – ethacrynic acid, bumetanide, furosemide and mersalyl - have been recognized to be active at a <u>medullary</u> diluting site on the thick ascending limb of Henle's loop. Thus, specific structure-function relationships do not appear to exist among diuretics except insofar as they are organic acids. But no one, I believe, would claim that all organic acids are diuretics, and conversely two diuretics, triamterene and amiloride, active at the far distal sodium/potassium exchange site clearly cannot be classified as organic acids.

However, molecular structures determining participation in the organic acid tubular transport system are clearly pertinent. The diuretic effect of mersalyl (<u>14</u>) and ethacrynic acid (<u>15</u>) appears to be due to inhibition by these drugs in the tubular lumen of active chloride transport in the thick ascending limb of Henle's loop. Similar data are available for furosemide <u>in vitro</u> (<u>16</u>), and in man (<u>17</u>); the diuretic response is determined by the amount of furosemide that reaches the renal tubule rather than the drug level in plasma (<u>18</u>). Similarly, in the dog, it has been found that those compounds which, administered in sufficient dose, inhibit renal transport of ticrynafen, also reduce ticrynafen natriuresis (<u>19</u>).

To add to the complexities facing the medicinal chemist synthesizing a new diuretic, is the observation that ticrynafen has a significant uricosuric activity. That an organic acid should have uricosuric activity is not totally unexpected. Any

list of uricosuric agents, from acetoheximide to zoxazolamine
will easily include 30 compounds of widely differing chemical
structure, the majority of which are organic acids. However,
weak organic bases such as zoxazolamine are also uricosuric. What
is unexpected is that orally active diuretics which should
increase uric acid excretion, generally cause a significant
uric acid retention, possibly due to their contraction of extracellular fluid volume (20) and/or inhibition of urate secretion.
      In the phosphate-mannitol infused mongrel dog, ticrynafen
at doses of 0.5 to 15 mg/kg intravenously, is natriuretic and
uricosuric (Table VII). Glomerular filtration rate was determined by the clearance of ^{3}H-inulin, and p-aminohippurate was
omitted from the infusion solution. The dogs were not urate
loaded. Under these conditions, ticrynafen was found to be
natriuretic and uricosuric, roughly equivalent in uricosuric
potency to probenecid. These data are in agreement with the
original reports of uricosuria induced in the mongrel dog,
reported by Beyer et al. (21) and by Sougin-Mibashan and Horwitz
(22).

TABLE VII

DIURETIC AND URICOSURIC ACTIVITY IN THE MONGREL DOG

Compound	Sodium* FE %	^{C}Ur* ml/min	Urate* FE %
Probenecid	0	+ 16.2	+ 31
10 mg/kg I.V.			
Hydrochlorothiazide	+ 5.3	− 2.3	− 1
0.5 mg/kg + 0.5 mg/kg/hr			
Ticrynafen			
1.5 mg/kg + 1.5 mg/kg/hr	+ 2.1	+ 8.7	+ 18
4 mg/kg I.V.	+ 4.2	+ 7.5	+ 17
10 mg/kg I.V.	+ 4.7	+ 9.8	+ 25
15 mg/kg I.V.	+ 8.5	+12.6	+ 22

* change from control

^{C}Ur = clearance of urate

      In man, ticrynafen is markedly uricosuric (Table VIII), the
fractional excretion of urate rising to a maximum in one volunteer of 75% of the filtered load. As a consequence of the
uricosuria, serum urate levels and, consequently, the filtered
load of urate to the kidney is sharply reduced. In contrast, the
ability of the orally active diuretics, especially the thiazides
and furosemide, to retain uric acid and increase the filtered
urate load is well recognized (23).

TABLE VIII

URICOSURIC ACTIVITY OF TICRYNAFEN IN HYDRATED
NORMAL MALE VOLUNTEERS

Volunteer		Dose mg	U_{Ur} V μg/min	C_{Ur}/C_{In} x 100
S-82	C	--	634	8.8
	E	500	2558	38.6
S-83	C	--	600	12.3
	E	500	2680	63.3
S-84	C	--	475	7.5
	E	500	2836	75.4
S-127	C	--	680	7.7
	E	1000	3173	58.8

Although researchers in the field of urate transport do not agree on the renal tubular site of urate reabsorption, a proximal site of urate transport is considered possible. Sulfinpyrazone, probenecid and aspirin are secreted by an organic acid secretory carrier located in the proximal tubule (24). Diamond and Meisel (25) have demonstrated that probenecid secretion is required for its uricosuric effect, and they have proposed that competition for binding at a urate-reabsorptive site on the tubular luminal surface may account for the effect of probenecid (26).

In the mongrel dog, competition with ticrynafen secretion reduced the uricosuric activity of ticrynafen as it reduced the natriuretic activity of the drug. Thus, increasingly a case may be made for the proximal transport of diuretics to act from the tubular lumen (19). It is a challenge to the medicinal chemist to fit his newly synthesized molecules to this renal transport system.

In summary, the data obtained in this study of ticrynafen clearly indicate that modification of chemical structures to obtain new diuretics requires the extensive participation of the physiologist.

Literature Cited

1. Burg, M. and Stoner, L., Ann. Rev. Physiol. (1976), 38, 37-45.

2. Goldberg, M., McCurdy, D. K., Foltz, E. L. and Bluemle, L. W., J. Clin. Invest. (1964), 43, 201-216.

3. Puschett, J. B. and Goldberg, M., J. Lab. Clin. Med. (1968), 71, 666-676.

4. Jayakumar, S. and Puschett, J. B., J. Pharm. Exptl. Therap. (1977), 201, 251-258.

5. Burg, M., "The Mechanism of Action of Diuretics in Renal

Tubules." Recent Advances Renal Physiol. Pharm., Ed., L. G. Wesson and G. M. Fanelli, University Park Press, (1974).
6. Beyer, K. H., Baer, J. E., Michaelson, J. K. and Russo, H. F., J. Pharm. Exptl. Therap. (1965), 147, 1-22.
7. Seldin, D. W., Eknoyan, G., Suki, W. N. and Rector, F. C., Ann. N. Y. Acad. Sci. (1966), 139, 328-343.
8. Clapp, J. R. and Robinson, R. R., Am. J. Physiol. (1968), 215, 228-235.
9. Baer, J. E., Michaelson, J. K., McKinstry, D. N. and Beyer, K. H., Proc. Soc. Exptl. Biol. Med. (1964), 115, 87-90.
10. Stote, R. M., Maass, A. R. Cherrill, D. A., Beg, M. M. A. and Alexander, F., J. Pharmacol. Clin. (Special Issue 1976), 19-27.
11. Goldberg, M., McCurdy, D., Foltz, E. and Bluemle, L., J. Clin. Invest. (1964), 43, 201-216.
12. Buckalew, V. M., Walker, B. R., Puschett, J. B. and Goldberg, M., J. Clin. Invest. (1970), 49, 2336-2344.
13. Seldin, D. W., Eknoyan, G., Suki, W. N. and Rector, F. C., Ann. N. Y. Acad. Sci. (1966), 139, 328-343.
14. Burg, M. and Green, N., Kidney Int. (1973), 4, 245-251.
15. Burg, M. and Green, N., Kidney Int. (1973), 4, 301-306.
16. Burg, M., Stoner, L., Cardinal, J. and Green, N., Am. J. Physiol. (1973), 225, 119-124.
17. Homeida, H., Roberts, C. and Branch, R. A., Clin. Pharm. Therap. (1977), 22, 402-409.
18. Honari, J., Blair, A. D. and Cutler, R. E., Clin. Pharm. Therap. (1977), 22, 395-401.
19. Maass, A. R. and Snow, I. B. To be published.
20. Steele, T. H. and Oppenheimer, S., Am. J. Physiol. (1969), 47, 564-574.
21. Beyer, K. H., Russo, H. F., Tillson, E. K., Miller, A. K., Verwey, W. F., Gass, S. R., Am. J. Physiol. (1951), 166, 625-640.
22. Sougin-Mibashan, R. and Horwitz, M., Lancet (1955), 1, 1191-1197.
23. Wyngaarten, J. B. and Kelley, W. N., "Drug-Induced Hyperuricemia and Gout" in Gout and Hyperuricemia, 369-370, Grune & Stratton (1976).
24. Tune, B. M., Burg, M. B. and Patlak, C. S., Am. J. Physiol. (1969), 217, 1057-1063.
25. Meisel, A. D. and Diamond, H. S., Arth. Rheum. (1977), 20, 128.
26. Diamond, H. S. and Meisel, A. D., Clin. Sci. Mol. Med. (1977), 53, 133-139.

RECEIVED August 21, 1978.

2-Aminomethylphenols: A New Class of Saluretic Agents

R. L. SMITH, E. M. SCHULTZ, G. E. STOKKER, and E. J. CRAGOE, JR.

Merck Sharp and Dohme Research Laboratories, West Point, PA 19486

A continuing search for new renal agents in our laboratories by screening carefully selected compounds for diuretic and saluretic activity in rats and dogs led to the discovery of 2-aminomethyl-3,4,6-trichlorophenol (Ia). The unusual structural features, attractive electrolyte excretion profile and saluretic potency of compound Ia relative to those of known diuretics (see Table I for an activity comparison) provided impetus for an extensive synthetic program. The data obtained facilitated the delineation of the structure-activity relationships for a variety of 2-aminomethylphenols and culminated in the development of 2-aminomethyl-4-(1,1-dimethylethyl)-6-iodophenol hydrochloride (MK-447). This compound was found to be a potent, high-ceiling salidiuretic agent with adjunctive antihypertensive and anti-inflammatory properties, and it is currently undergoing clinical evaluation. This report is a preliminary account (1) of the highlights of our research on this new class of saluretic agents.

TABLE I.   Relative Saluretic Activities[a]

Compound	Species (Admin. Route)	
	Rat (p.o.)	Dog (i.v.)
Ia	3	4
Hydrochlorothiazide	2	2
Furosemide	3	5
Ethacrynic Acid	0	5

[a]Presented as scores; assay protocols are described in the text, and scoring criteria are presented in Tables II and III.

0-8412-0464-0/78/47-083-**093**$08.25/0

SALIDIURETIC ACTIVITY ASSAYS

The structure-activity relationships (vide infra) in this study were determined by evaluating each synthetic compound for salidiuretic activity in two animal species, the rat and the dog. A brief description of each assay protocol is given below along with the system used to score the biological results.

Oral Rat Assay - Female rats (Charles River, 150-170 g), housed in metabolism cages in groups of three rats per cage, were maintained overnight on a sugar diet with water ad libitum. At the time of the test, each animal was given the test compound orally either as a solution or suspension in 5 ml of water. Urine was collected over the 0-5 hr interval in graduated cylinders and subsequently analyzed for sodium, potassium and chloride content by standard methodology. The saluretic response was scored from 0 to 6 according to the natriuretic criteria indicated in Table II.

TABLE II.   Scoring System for Oral Rat Assay

| Score | μEq Na^+/cage, dose in mg/kg | | | | |
	1	5	16.5	50	81
0				0.3	0.3
$\pm$			0.4	0.7	0.9
1		0.3	0.5	1.2	1.5
2		0.4	0.6	1.8	2.4
3		0.5	1.4	2.4	2.9
4		1.4	2.7	3.3	
5	0.7	2.6	3.3	3.6	
6	2.1	3.6	4.2	3.9	

Intravenous Dog Assay - Conditioned female mongrel dogs, weighing approximately 20 kg in the postabsorptive state, were starved overnight and then given 500 ml of water orally 1 hr before induction of anesthesia with sodium pentobarbital (30 mg/kg, i.v.). After inducing anesthesia, each dog was prepared with an indwelling bladder catheter and primed with creatinine (4 g as a 10% solution in water) administered s.c. in multiple injection sites. To ensure uniform hydration and urine production, 1.5 ml/kg of an isoosmotic pH 7.4 phosphate buffer solution (20 mg phosphate/kg) was given i.v. as a priming injection prior to initiation of clearance studies and 3 ml/min of an isoosmotic pH 7.4 buffer containing 4% mannitol (6.9 mg phosphate/min) was infused during the experiment. At the start of timed clearances, the urinary bladder was emptied and replicate 15-min urine collections were made with venous blood samples being drawn at the midpoint of each period. Following this control phase, the test compound was administered i.v. stat (i.e., over a 5 min period) at 5 mg/kg. Urine was collected over replicate 15 min periods for 2 hr and subsequently assayed for electrolyte content by standard methodology. The average rate of natriuresis determined for the two highest consecutive 15 min collection periods was used to score the saluretic response from 0 to 5 on the basis of the sodium excretion rates indicated in Table III.

TABLE III.   Scoring System for Intravenous Dog Assay

Score	μEq Na$^+$/min at 5 mg/kg I.V. Stat
0	0-99
$\pm$	active above 5 mg/kg
1	100-399
2	400-599
3	600-799
4	800-899
5	900

STRUCTURE-ACTIVITY RELATIONSHIPS

The initial phase of this investigation was directed toward determination of the biological consequences resulting from reorientation and structural modification of the hydroxyl (phenolic) and aminomethyl groups in compound Ia. As is shown in Table IV, orientation of these functional groups in either a meta (Compound Ib) or para (Compound Ic) relationship with concomitant positional interchange of the aminomethyl moiety with either the 3- or 4-chloro substituent resulted in ablation of activity. Hence, these results established the importance of maintaining an ortho relationship between the hydroxyl and aminomethyl groups.

TABLE IV.   Orientation Effects

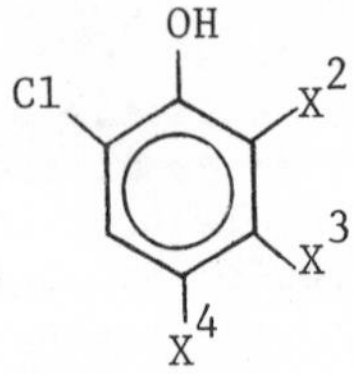

(I)

| | | | | Saluretic Score | |
Compd.	X^2	X^3	X^4	Rat	Dog
Ia	CH_2NH_2	Cl	Cl	3	4
b	Cl	CH_2NH_2	Cl	0	0
c	Cl	Cl	CH_2NH_2	0	0

The effects of N-substitution on saluretic activity were explored next and are tabulated for a representative series of structures in Table V. As the data indicate, alkylation of the amino group proved to be detrimental to activity as did acylation, with exception of N-trifluoroacetylation. In the latter case, the activity elicited upon oral administration of compound IIg in the rat most likely resulted from its in vivo hydrolysis to the active precursor, compound Ia. Indeed, the observed facile conversion of trifluoroacetamide IIg to amine Ia under mild hydrolytic conditions (e.g., 20°C, pH 8, 30 min) in vitro is consistent with this viewpoint.

Meadow, et al (2, 3) have reported some of the biological activities displayed by a series of tertiary amines of general formula III; compound IIIa was identified as the most active diuretic member of the series. In our laboratories, compound IIIa was found to be inactive in both the rat and dog diuretic assays under a variety of test conditions. This result is interesting in view of the activity, albeit weak, displayed by tertiary amine IIc.

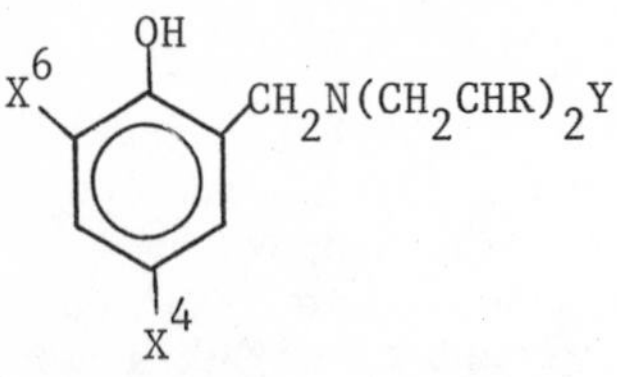

IIIa, R=H; Y=O;
X^4=$CH_2CH=CH_2$;
X^6=OCH_3

Alteration of the aminomethyl group, e.g., by α-substitution (Compound IVa), homologation (Compound IVb) or simultaneous α-substitution and homologation (Compound IVc), led to substantial diminution in activity as demonstrated in Table VI. Furthermore,

TABLE V

Effects of N-Substitution

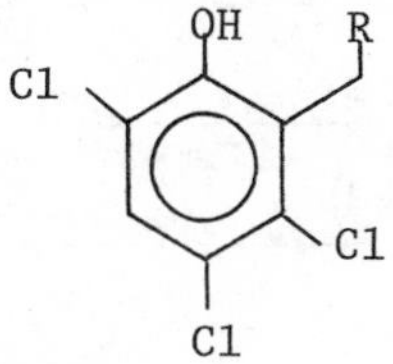

(II)

Compd	R	Saluretic Score	
		Rat	Dog
IIa	$NHCH_3$	1	
b	$N(CH_3)_2$	2	0
c	$N(CH_2CH_2)_2O$	±	1
d	$N(CH_3)CH_2$⎯⎰O⎱	1	1
e	NHCHO	0	0
f	$NHCOCH_2Cl$	1	0
g	$NHCOCF_3$	3	
h	$NHCOCH_2NH_2$	±	1

the corresponding salicylalcohol (Compound IVd), salicylaldehyde
(Compound IVe) and salicylic acid (Compound IVf) analogs of
compound Ia were devoid of demonstrable saluretic activity.

TABLE VI. Effects of Aminomethyl Group Alteration

$$OH$$

(structure IV: benzene ring bearing OH, three Cl substituents, and X^2) (IV)

Compd.	X^2	Saluretic Score	
		Rat	Dog
IVa	$CH(CH_3)NH_2$	$\pm$	
b	$CH_2CH_2NH_2$	1	1
c	$CH(OH)CH_2NH_2$	0	1
d	CH_2OH	0	0
e	CHO	0	0
f	CO_2H	0	0

To complete the preliminary SAR studies, the effects of
hydroxyl group modification were determined; the results are
presented in Table VII. As the data indicate, both O-alkylation
(e.g., as in compounds Va-c) and replacement of OH by NH_2 resulted
in structures with marginal saluretic activity. These results
coupled with those presented previously (vide supra) indicated
that: (a) the ortho orientation of the hydroxyl and aminomethyl
groups (i.e., as in salicylamine) should be maintained, and that
(b) these two functional groups must remain unsubstituted. Ac-
cordingly, the effects of nuclear substitution, both singularly
and multiply, were investigated in a systematic manner as an
approach to improving saluretic activity.

Data for a representative series of monosubstituted salicylamines (Compound VI) bearing substituents in the 4-position are
shown in Table VIII. Although salicylamine itself (Compound IVa)
is devoid of demonstrable salidiuretic activity, introduction of a
chloro group in the 4-position (Compound VIb) imparts weak saluretic properties which are maintained upon replacement of the
chloro group by lower alkyl groups up to and including a three
carbon straight chain, with or without α-branching. However,
introduction of the n-butyl group in the 4-position is not tolerated, since compound VIf did not exhibit demonstrable activity
in either the rat or the dog assay.

TABLE VII

Effects of Phenol Group Modification

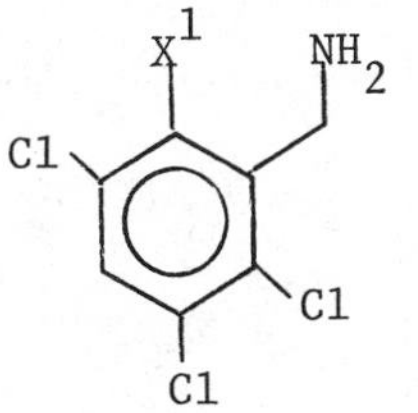

(V)

Compd	X^1	Saluretic Score	
		Rat	Dog
Va	OCH_3	$\pm$	0
b	$OCH_2CO_2C_2H_5$	1	0
c	OCH_2CO_2H	$\pm$	
d	NH_2	$\pm$	0

TABLE VIII.   Effects of Nuclear Monosubstitution

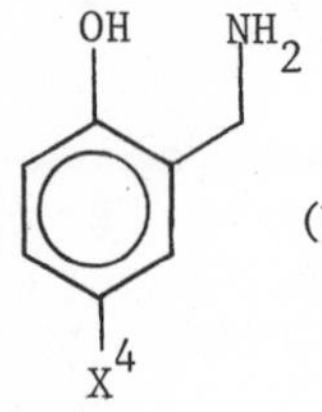

Compd.	X^4	Saluretic Score	
		Rat	Dog
VIa	H	0	0
b	Cl	1	1
c	C_2H_5	1	1
d	$C(CH_3)_3$	1	
e	$CH(CH_3)C_2H_5$	1	0
f	$(CH_2)_3CH_3$	0	0

Appropriate nuclear disubstitution led to marked enhancement of saluretic activity as indicated by the results tabulated in Table IX. The dichloro derivatives (Compounds VIIa-c) illustrate the importance of the 4,6-disubstitution pattern, i.e., VIIb is more active than the other positional isomers. This observation, coupled with the information gained from the monosubstituted series, prompted preparation of compounds VIId-i. Replacement of the 4-chloro group in compound VIIb with lower alkyl groups led to markedly improved activity which peaked in potency with the introduction of a 4-(1,1-dimethylethyl) moiety, i.e., compound VIIi. Interestingly, the 6-chloro, 6-bromo and 6-iodo derivatives (i.e., compounds VIIi, VIIk and VIIl, respectively) elicit marked salidiuretic responses, whereas, the 6-fluoro analog (Compound VIIj) is considerably less active. As will be discussed subsequently, the pronounced antihypertensive properties of MK-447 (Compound VIIl) served to distinguish it from a subseries of nearly equipotent saluretic agents which emerged during the course of this investigation. Finally, it should be noted that compound VIIm, the primary amine analog of compound IIIa (vide supra), displayed good activity in both rats and dogs.

The influences of nuclear trisubstitution on saluretic activity are presented in Table X for a group of compounds of the general structure VIII. It is noteworthy that shifting the 3-chloro substituent in compound Ia to the 5-position (i.e., to afford compound VIIIa) resulted in slightly improved activity in the dog; whereas, movement of the 6-chloro group in Ia to the

TABLE IX

Effects of Nuclear Disubstitution

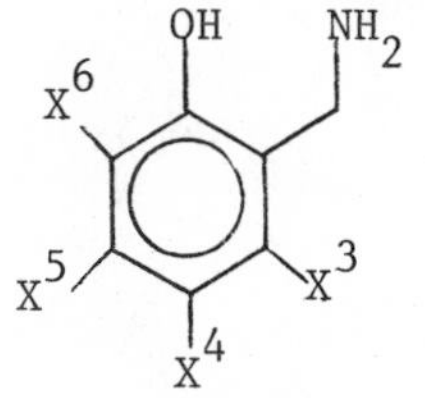

(VII)

Compd	X^3	X^4	X^5	X^6	Saluretic Score	
					Rat	Dog
VIIa	Cl	Cl	H	H	1	1
b	H	Cl	H	Cl	2	$\pm$
c	Cl	H	H	Cl	0	1
d	H	CH_3	H	Cl	2	1
e	H	C_2H_5	H	Cl	4	5
f	H	$(CH_2)_2CH_3$	H	Cl	4	5
g	H	$CH_2CH(CH_3)_2$	H	Cl	3	2
h	H	$CH(CH_3)C_2H_5$	H	Cl	5	4
i	H	$C(CH_3)_3$	H	Cl	6	5
j	H	$C(CH_3)_3$	H	F	4	5
k	H	$C(CH_3)_3$	H	Br	6	5
l[a]	H	$C(CH_3)_3$	H	I	6	5
m	H	$CH_2CH=CH_2$	H	OCH_3	3	2

[a] Compound VIIl = MK-447

5-position (i.e., to form compound VIIIb) diminished activity in
the dog while marginally enhancing activity in the rat. Furthermore, introduction of electron donating substituents (e.g., methyl
and methoxy groups) in the 6-position, as in compounds VIIIf and
VIIIg, proved to reduce activity in both test species.

TABLE X.   Effects of Nuclear Trisubstitution

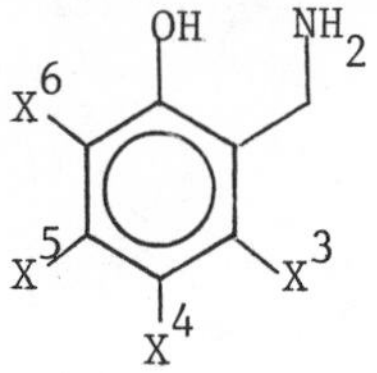

(VIII)

Compd.	X^3	X^4	X^5	X^6	Saluretic Score	
					Rat	Dog
Ia	Cl	Cl	H	Cl	3	4
VIIIa	H	Cl	Cl	Cl	4	4
b	Cl	Cl	Cl	H	4	2
c	F	Cl	H	Cl	4	4
d	Cl	Cl	H	CF_3	4	2
e	CH_3	CH_3	H	Cl	3	2
f	CH_3	CH_3	H	CH_3	2	1
g	Cl	Cl	H	OCH_3	1	1
h	OH	Cl	H	Cl	1	0

Finally, the data recorded in Table XI illustrate the
effects of nuclear tetrasubstitution on activity. These data
reveal several interesting SAR trends. First, although replacement of the 3- and 5-chloro substituents of tetrachloro derivative
IXa with methyl groups resulted in greatly enhanced activity
in the dog, most surprisingly, the interchange of chloro and
methyl substituents (i.e., conversion of Compound IXb to compound
IXc) totally abolished activity. These results indicate that
both steric and electronic effects contribute substantially
in determining the saluretic efficacy of these structures.
Reinforcement for the importance of these effects is provided
by activity comparisons of structures IXe with IXf and IXg
with IXh. Diminution of activity accompanies replacement

of a chloro substituent with a methyl group (electronic effect) in the first instance and reflects the rather stringent steric requirements for substituents in the 3-position in the second instance. Secondly, the results tabulated for compounds IXb, IXi and IXk suggest that, whereas the methyl groups in the 3- and 5-positions can be replaced with methoxy groups with maintenance of activity, their replacement with ethoxy moieties substantially reduces activity. The latter result is in accord with the steric restraints discussed above for substituents in the 3-position. Furthermore, it should be noted that compounds IXg and IXi display saluretic activities which are essentially of the same magnitude as those of the 4-(1,1-dimethylethyl)-6-halosalicylamines (i.e., VIIi, VIIk and VIIl) cited earlier.

TABLE XI. Effects of Nuclear Tetrasubstitution

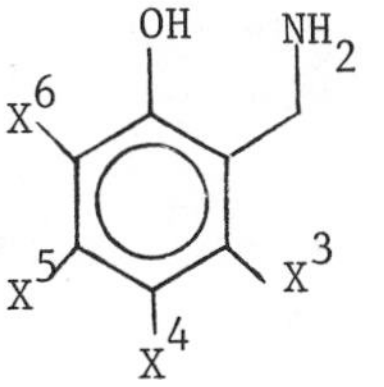

(IX)

Compd.	X^3	X^4	X^5	X^6	Saluretic Score Rat	Saluretic Score Dog
IXa	Cl	Cl	Cl	Cl	4	1
b	CH_3	Cl	CH_3	Cl	4	5
c	Cl	CH_3	Cl	CH_3	0	0
d	CH_3	Br	CH_3	Br	4	5
e	CH_3	CH_3	Cl	Cl	5	2
f	CH_3	CH_3	CH_3	CH_3	3	1
g	CH_3	Cl	C_2H_5	Cl	5	5
h	C_2H_5	Cl	CH_3	Cl	1	1
i	OCH_3	Cl	OCH_3	Cl	5	5
j	OCH_3	Cl	OCH_3	Br	5	3
k	OC_2H_5	Cl	OC_2H_5	Cl	3	0

In summary, these SAR studies indicate that saluretic activity is elicited by 2-aminomethylphenols which are appropriately
substituted with a hydrogen, methyl or methoxy group in the
3-position, a halo or lower alkyl (i.e., ≤ three carbon straight
chain, preferably α-branched) moiety in the 4-position, a hydrogen
or lower alkyl (or alkoxy) substituent in the 5-position and a
iodo, bromo or chloro group in the 6-position, the optimal substituent combinations and patterns being determined by the cited
SARs.

CHEMISTRY

The two general synthetic routes which were most frequently
used to prepare the salicylamine derivatives studied during the
course of this investigation are summarized in Scheme I. The first
route involves acid-catalyzed nuclear amidoalkylation of an
appropriately substituted phenol (Compound X) with an N-hydroxy-
methylamide, $RCONHCH_2OH$ ($R=CH_3$, CH_2Cl, CCl_3, CF_3 or C_6H_5), to give
an N-acylsalicylamine of general formula XI. Subsequent hydro-
lytic N-deacylation of compound XI followed by halogenation
affords the target product. The second route involves the same
steps but in an altered order, i.e., halogenation of phenol X to
give an o-halophenol of general structure XII followed by amidoalkylation and hydrolysis. In both sequences, the key amido-
methylation step is accomplished readily via the Tscherniac-
Einhorn reaction (4). The choice of the proper reaction sequence,
as well as optimum conditions (i.e., $RCONHCH_2OH$, acid catalyst,
reaction medium, etc.) for introducing the aminomethyl moiety, is
governed primarily by the chemical nature and directing influences
of the substituents X^3, X^4 and X^5. The importance of selecting
the proper acid catalyst and reaction medium to control the
amidoalkylation step is demonstrated in equation 1.

Scheme I

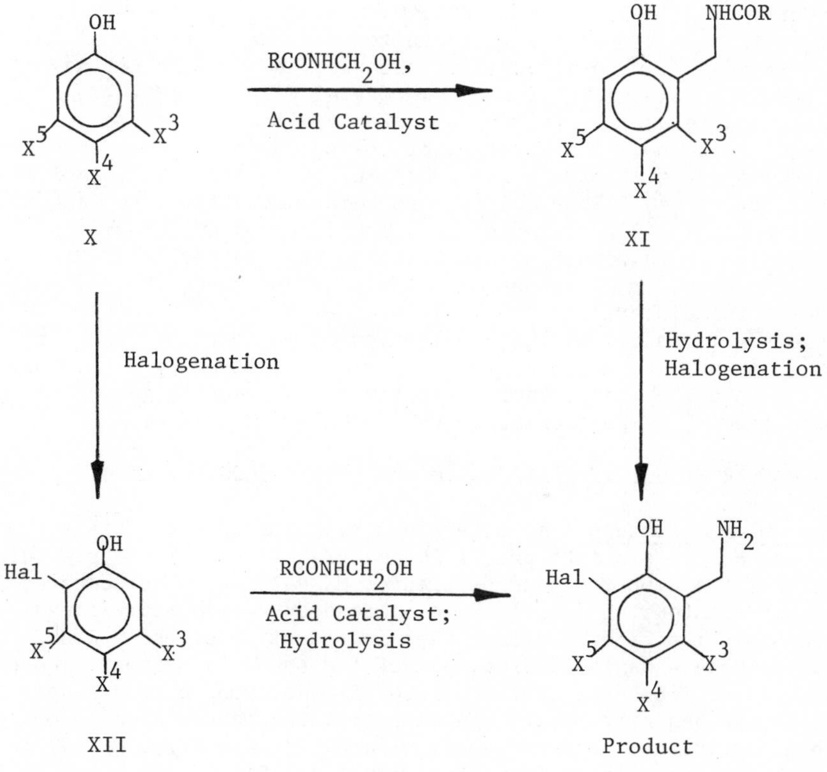

The desired amide (Compound XIa) is formed in good yield (60-
70%) when HOAc-H$_2$SO$_4$ (9:1) is used, whereas, the use of H$_2$SO$_4$
alone leads to extensive diamidomethylation (diamide XIII), even
when equimolar quantities of phenol Xa and N-hydroxymethylchloro-
acetamide are employed.

Application of these general synthetic routes to the elabo-
ration of MK-447 (5) from 4-(1,1-dimethylethyl)phenol (Compound
Xb) is shown in Figure 1. The reaction sequence, Xb ——>XIb ——>
XIV ——>MK-447, is the preferred synthetic pathway for preparing
large quantities of MK-447 and can be accomplished routinely in
50% overall yield. Since the 6-iodo substituent is introduced
under very mild conditions (ICl, 0.5N HCl, 20°C) in the terminal
step, this sequence is ideally suited for the synthesis of
$\angle^{131}$I$\angle$7-MK-447. The alternative pathway, Xb ——>XIIb (either
directly or stepwise via chloromercurial XIIa) ——>MK-447, although quite useful, is less satisfactory than the former as
discussed below. The intermediate o-iodophenol XIIb is somewhat
deactivated to electrophilic substitution relative to phenol Xa
and, therefore, XIIb requires more acidic conditions to facilitate
the Tscherniac-Einhorn reaction. The stronger acid medium is
conducive to deiodination and leads to reduced yields of MK447.
Nevertheless, the alternative pathway proved to be the route of
choice for elaborating MK-447 labeled with a 2-$\angle^{14}$C$\angle$7-aminomethyl
moiety. In this instance, conversion of o-iodophenol XIIb to
$\angle^{14}$C$\angle$7-MK-447 was achieved in 35% overall yield using N-(hydroxy-
$\angle^{14}$C$\angle$7-methyl)chloroacetamide which was conveniently generated in
situ from $\angle^{14}$C$\angle$7-paraformaldehyde and chloroacetamide.

MOLECULAR STRUCTURE, METABOLISM AND PHARMACOLOGY OF MK-447

Molecular Structure - As determined by potentiometric titration in
water, MK-447 exhibits pKa$_1$ 7.25 and pKa$_2$ 10.75. These pKa values
reflect the amphoteric properties of MK-447 and, when compared
with those (pKa$_{1,2}$ 8.4, 10.5) displayed by 2-aminomethylphenol
hydrochloride, they indicate that introduction of the 6-iodo
substituent enhances the acidity of the phenolic hydroxyl group
or, viewed from a different perspective, serves to reduce net
molecular basicity, i.e., monodeprotonation occurs at a lower pH.
When partitioned between 1-octanol and pH 7.4 buffer, MK-447 is
localized essentially quantitatively (ca. 99%) in the lipid phase.
The free base form of MK-447, readily liberated from MK-447 by
neutralization with weak bases such as ammonia and sodium bicarbonate, is very soluble in non-polar organic solvents and relatively insoluble in aqueous media. The limited water solubility
of MK-447 free base suggests that it has appreciable zwitterionic
character in water. Indeed, the validity of this suggestion was
confirmed by determining the effects of pH on λ_{max} for MK-447 in
water. The bathochromic shift from 285 to 309 mμ which accompanies
phenoxide formation (i.e., ArOH ——>ArO$^-$) was observed at pH 6.
Hence, the observed solubility characteristics of MK-447 free base

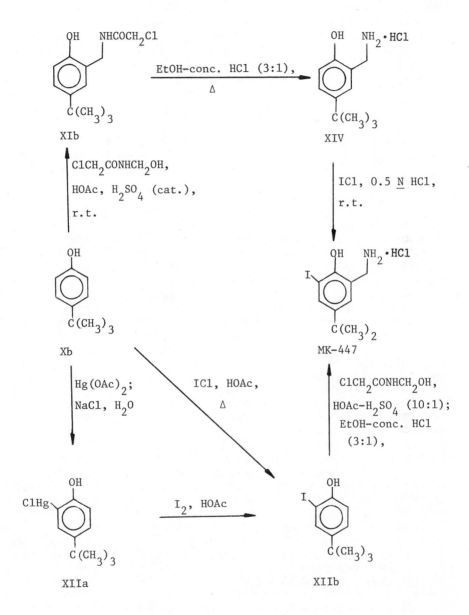

Figure 1. Synthetic routes to MK-447

reflect its unique ability to adjust molecular polarity in a
solvent-dependent manner as illustrated in equation 2. This
process should be quite facile since, a priori, minimal energy
would be required to effect the depicted intramolecular proton
transfer.

(Eq. 2)

"Uncharged Form"   "Zwitterion"

    Examination of the lowest energy ground state conformation of
compound VIIi, calculated by the CNDO/2 formalism (6) and presented as an ORTEP projection (7) in Figure 2, affords additional
insight into the physicochemical properties cited above. First,
the plane formed by the Cl-C6-Cl-O-H$_a$ atom array is coplanar with
the aromatic ring and the phenolic hydrogen atom (H$_a$) is hydrogen
bonded to the chloro substituent. This result is in accord with
the recent demonstration of intramolecular hydrogen bonding in
o-halophenols, including 2-iodophenols, by Kollman et al (8).
Furthermore, although the aminomethyl group is situated substantially out of the plane of the ring (θ = 45°), a second
intramolecular hydrogen bond exists between H$_b$ of the amino group
and the phenolic oxygen atom. The solid state structure of MK-447
free base, determined by the single crystal X-ray crystallographic
technique, is in reasonable agreement with the calculated ground-
state structure of compound VIIi. A comparison of these structures, shown by their superimposition (i.e., one over the other)
in Figure 3, indicates that they differ in two respects: (a)
compound VIIi contains a H$_a$...Cl, whereas, the -OH$_a$ group in
MK-447 free base is not intramolecularly hydrogen bonded; instead,
it is directed below and perpendicular to the plane of the aromatic ring and (b) the size of the dihedral angle θ (45° vs. 53°)
is minimally different. The first structural difference is
somewhat surprising and may well reflect the inherent difficulties
associated with accurately locating a hydrogen atom proximate to
an iodo substituent by X-ray crystallography. The minor difference in θ could either reflect the crystal packing forces in
the solid state or stem from the well-known overestimation of
attractive forces between non-bonded atoms by the CNDO/2 method
(9). In any event, the substitution of iodo and aminomethyl
groups vicinally to the hydroxyl moiety facilitates intramolecular
hydrogen bonding which, coupled with the presence of a 4-(1,1-
dimethylethyl) substituent, imparts substantial lipophilicity to
MK-447 free base. Likewise, this nuclear substitution pattern is

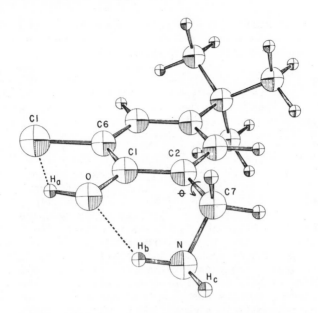

Figure 2. *The lowest energy ground state conformation of compound VIIi, the 6-chloro analog of MK-447 free base. This conformation, presented as an ORTEP projection, was calculated by the CNDO/2 semiempirical technique.*

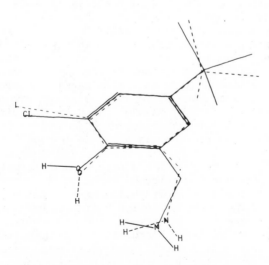

Figure 3. *Comparison of the x-ray structure of MK-447 free base (dotted lines) with the CNDO/2-calculated lowest energy ground state conformation of 6-chloro analog VIIi (solid lines)*

conducive to zwitterion formation in aqueous media and, thereby,
severely limits the solubility of MK-447 free base, but not that
of the parent hydrochloride, in water.

Metabolism - Studies (10) in rats, dogs and man indicate that
orally administered $\angle^{14}C\angle$-MK-447 is rapidly absorbed, metabolized
and excreted. Peak plasma drug levels were observed within 1 to 2
hr post drug administration in all three species; at this time,
the parent drug accounted for ca. 15% of the total $\angle^{14}C\angle$-radio-
activity in human plasma and ca. 5% of that in rat and dog plasma.
The half-life of drug-related $\angle^{14}C\angle$radioactivity in the plasma was
about 7.5 hr in man and dogs and 1 hr in rats. In each of these
species, the principle route of drug elimination (primarily as
metabolites XV and XVI, vide infra) was via the urine, whereas,
the feces constituted the minor pathway for drug excretion.
    As depicted in Scheme II, MK-447 is metabolized in rats and
dogs almost exclusively to the corresponding O-sulfate ester
(Compound XV). The major human metabolite of MK-447 has been
isolated and tentatively assigned structure XVI, the N-glucuronide
derivative of MK-447. The minor human metabolite corresponds to
O-sulfate ester XV. The assignment of structure XV to the major
rat and dog metabolite was confirmed by direct comparison of the
isolated metabolite with an authentic sample of 2-amino-
methyl-4-(1,1-dimethylethyl)-6-iodophenyl hydrogen sulfate which
was synthesized by the O-sulfation process presented in Scheme II.
    It should be noted that compound XV displays marked sali-
diuretic activity in both rats (saluretic score = 3) and dogs
(saluretic score = 5). In view of the data presented in Table VII
(vide supra) for O-substituted salicylamines Va-c, the observed
activity after administration of O-sulfate ester XV suggests that
O-desulfation occurs at the proper site in vivo, liberating MK-447
in agreement with the widely-accepted principle of microscopic
reversibility, at least as it applies to enzymatic transforma-
tions. Hence, although ultimately eliminated via urinary and
fecal excretion, metabolite XV may well serve in vivo as both a
depot and a pro-drug form of MK-447. Finally, in spite of its
structural similarity to thyroxine, MK-447 does not undergo
detectable deiodination either in vitro or in vivo.

Pharmacology (11) - Orally administered in both normotensive and
spontaneously hypertensive rats, MK-447 displayed marked saluretic
and diuretic effects which were rapid in onset and relatively
modest in duration, the major action having occurred within the
first 5 hrs. A comparison of the salidiuretic activities of
MK-447, furosemide and hydrochlorothiazide in normotensive rats is
presented in Figures 4, 5 and 6. For those renal parameters
measured, this comparison demonstrates that (a) the ceiling
effects of MK-447 exceed those of furosemide and hydrochlorothiazide and (b) MK-447 is significantly more potent than furosemide. A precise comparison of the relative potencies of MK-447

Scheme II

Metabolism of MK-447

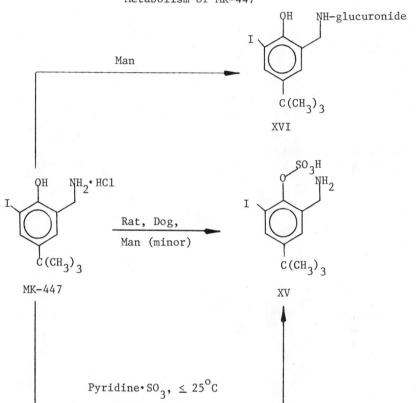

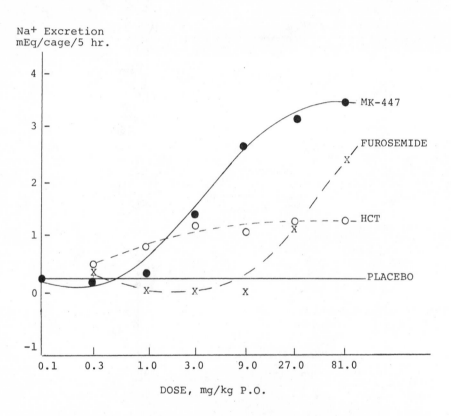

Figure 4.   Dose–response regression lines for the natriuretic effects of orally-administered MK-447, furosemide, and hydrochlorothiazide in normotensive rats over a five-hr period.   The data points are average values determined per cage for six to nine cages (three rats per cage of each drug.   The placebo values for the same period were: Na⁺, 0.28; K⁺, 0.16; and Cl⁻, 0.25 mEq/cage, and urine volume, 28 mL/cage.

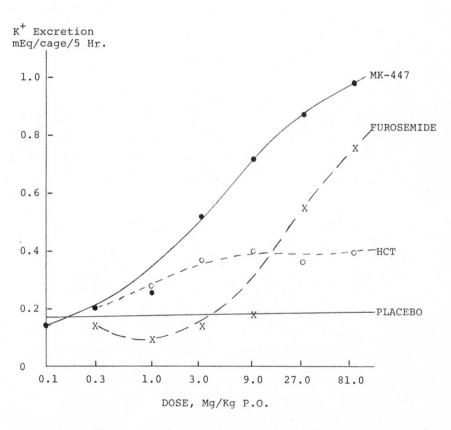

K⁺ Excretion
mEq/cage/5 Hr.

Figure 5. Dose–response regression lines for the kaliuretic effects of orally-administered MK-447, furosemide, and hydrochlorothiazide in normotensive rats over a five-hr period. The data points are average values determined per cage for six to nine cages (three rats per cage) at each dose of each drug. The placebo values for the same period were: Na⁺, 0.28; K⁺, 0.16; and Cl⁻, 0.25 mEq/cage, and urine volume, 28 mL/cage.

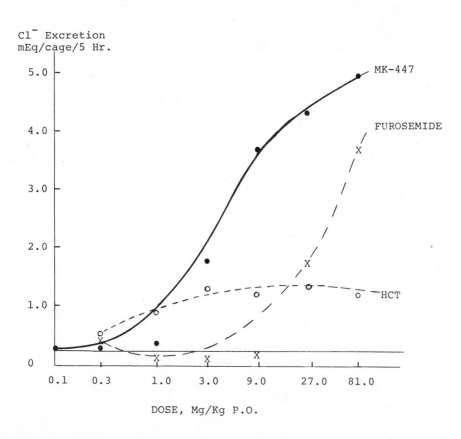

Figure 6. Dose–response regression lines for the chloruretic effects of orally-adminis-tered MK-447, furosemide, and hydrochlorothiazide in normotensive rats over a five-hr period. The data points are average values determined per cage for six to nine cages (three rats per cage) at each dose of each drug. The placebo values for the same period were: Na⁺, 0.28; K⁺, 0.16; and Cl⁻, 0.25 mEq/cage, and urine volume, 28 mL/cage.

and hydrochlorothiazide is precluded by the lack of slope parallelism in their dose-response regression lines.

Evidence that the salidiuretic activity of MK-447 may relate to its ability to enhance kidney levels of PGE has been provided by Kuehl, et al. (12, 13) who showed that this drug has the ability to enhance the synthesis of PGEs in ram seminal vesicular microsomes and in incubating kidney slices. A typical experiment demonstrating the ability of MK-447 to facilitate the conversion of arachidonic acid to PGE$_2$ is shown in Figure 8. The mechanistic details for this action of MK-447 have been described (12, 14).

Support for the concept that the salidiuretic action of MK-447 relates to PG production is provided by the finding that treatment of rats with indomethacin (2 mg/kg p.o.) 1 hr prior to dosing with MK-447 affected both electrolyte excretion and urine volumes as shown in Table XII. This effect of indomethacin on the salidiuretic action of MK-447 was dose-dependent, since pretreatment with a lower dose (1 mg/kg p.o.) of indomethacin did not significantly affect the potency of MK-447. On the other hand, at a dose of 4 mg/kg p.o., indomethacin substantially reduced both the saluretic and diuretic effects of MK-447. Furthermore, indomethacin (4 mg/kg p.o.) alone marginally reduced rat urine volumes, which suggests that the observed effect of indomethacin pretreatment may be due only partially to a specific antagonism of the diuretic actions of MK-447.

The salidiuretic effects of MK-447, furosemide and hydrochlorothiazide given p.o. in unanesthetized dogs are compared in Table XIII. At each of the doses studied, MK-447 displayed saluretic and diuretic effects greater in magnitude than those of either furosemide or hydrochlorothiazide. As observed in rats, MK-447 elicited slightly more chloruresis than natriuresis in dogs. Kaliuresis was increased significantly by each of the three drugs. In anesthetized dogs, dose-related increases in electrolyte excretion and urinary volumes resulted from MK-447 given i.v. over the entire 0.1 to 25 mg/kg dose range. The Na$^+$/K$^+$ excretion ratio approached 14 at the highest dose (25 mg/kg i.v.).

When evaluated in spontaneously hypertensive (SH) rats, MK-447 (dose $\geq$ 0.312 mg/kg p.o.) exhibited antihypertensive activity. At doses of 1.25 and 5 mg/kg p.o., the antihypertensive effects of MK-447 were rapid in onset (within 1 hr), pronounced in potency and prolonged in duration (24 hr). In addition, the antihypertensive activity of MK-447 in SH rats was maintained upon repeated oral administration at 0.312 mg/kg as demonstrated in Table XIV. Under conditions where MK-447 (0.312 mg/kg p.o.) produced a pronounced antihypertensive response, furosemide at 20 mg/kg p.o. exhibited no hypotensive effect.

Evidence which suggests that the renal prostaglandins, in addition to their possible contribution to the salidiuretic

116 DIURETIC AGENTS

TABLE XII

Antagonism of the Saluretic and Diuretic Effects
of MK-447 by Indomethacin Pretreatment[a] in
Normotensive Rats

Treatment	Dose (mg/kg p.o.)	Excretion Values[b], 0-5 Hr Period			
		Na^+ (mEq)	K^+ (mEq)	Cl^- (mEq)	Urine Vol (ml)
Placebo	0	0.28	0.16	0.25	28
MK-447	9	2.70	0.77	3.64	44
MK-447	27	3.19	0.88	4.35	47
MK-447	81	3.51	0.99	4.89	47
MK-447 + Indomethacin	9 2	2.52	0.85	3.59	42
MK-447 + Indomethacin	27 2	2.97	0.97	4.24	45
MK-447 + Indomethacin	81 2	3.25	1.02	4.70	43

[a]Pretreatment 1 hr prior to dosing with MK-447. [b]Average values
per cage, 3 rats per cage.

TABLE XIII

Saluretic and Diuretic Effects of Orally Administered
MK-447 (MK), Furosemide (F) and
Hydrochlorothiazide (HCT) in Unanesthetized Dogs

Dose (mg/kg)	Excretion Values[a], 0-24 hr. Period											
	Na^+ (mEq)			K^+ (mEq)			Cl^- (mEq)			Urine Vol (ml)		
	MK	F	HCT	MK	F	HCT	MK	F	HCT	MK	F	HCT
0.2	10			6			12			260		
0.3	16	12	9	7	6	5	17	12	11	330	510	375
0.5			15			8			15			440
0.6	25			11			36			540		
1		22	19		8	8		25	26		660	800
1.3	38			19			46			570		
1.8	42			16			52			700		
2	50			17			73			890		
3		37			10			44			725	
5	59		24	18		10	77		31	960		590
10		57	26		18	12		69	31		1035	760

[a] Average values determined per dog for 3 to 47 dogs at each dose of each drug. The placebo values for the same period were: Na^+, 4.8; K^+, 6.3; and Cl^-, 6.3 mEq/dog and urine volume, 210 ml/dog.

TABLE XIV

Antihypertensive Activity of MK-447 Administered
Orally in SH Rats of the Wistar-Okamoto Strain

Group No. (No. of Rats)	Treatment	Day	Mean Arterial Pressure (mmHg $\pm$ SE)[a], Hr after Treatment			
			0	4	12	24
1 (17)	Saline 2 ml/kg p.o.	1	178+4	180+4	174+3	172+3
		2		173+4	171+3	171+3
		3		171+2	170+2	173+2
2 (5)	MK-447[b]	1	185+3	163+5	166+7	167+7
		2		157+7	161+6	156+5
		3		157+4	159+3	181+4

[a]Arterial pressure was recorded in unanesthetized male rats of
290 to 350 g body weight and 30 to 40 weeks age by a direct
technique involving cannulation of the caudal artery. [b]MK-447
(0.312 mg/kg) was administered p.o. in water in volumes of
2 ml/kg daily for 3 days.

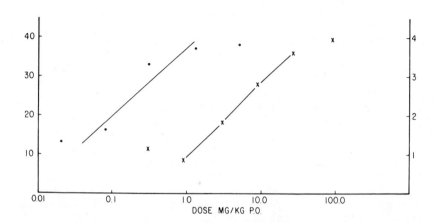

Figure 7. Dose–response regression lines for the effects of MK-447 on the mean arterial pressure and Na⁺ excretion in spontaneously hypertensive rats. The data points for decreases in mean arterial pressure are average values per rat for four to six rats per dose; the data points for Na⁺ excretion are average values per cage determined for nine cages (three rats per cage) at each dose.

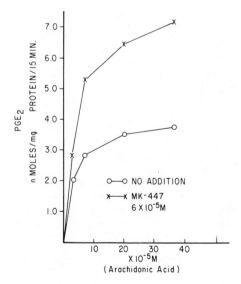

Figure 8. The stimulatory effects of MK-447 on the biosynthesis of PGE₂ in ram seminal vesicular microsomes as a function of substrate concentration

effects of MK-447 (<u>vide</u> <u>supra</u>), may also play a role in mediating
the antihypertensive activity of MK-447 emerged from studies in
SH rats. In this test species, the marked antihypertensive
effects elicited by 0.078, 0.312 and 1.25 mg/kg p.o. doses of
MK-447 were seriously attenuated by the oral coadministration of
either indomethacin (1.25 mg/kg) or aspirin (20 mg/kg). Interestingly, MK-447 displayed no hypotensive activity in normotensive
Wistar-Kyoto rats at doses up to 20 mg/kg p.o. Of even greater
pharmacological interest was the observation that MK-447 exhibited antihypertensive activity in SH rats at subdiuretic doses,
i.e., at doses ten-fold lower than those required for diuresis as
shown by the dose-response regression lines in Figure 7.

The results cited above indicate that, at least in SH rats,
the antihypertensive activity of MK-447 is not solely dependent
on its diuretic activity. Further support for this view emerges
upon examination of the relative saluretic and antihypertensive
activities recorded in Table XV for a series of salicylamine
derivatives. Although compounds IXg, IXi, VIIi, VIIk and MK-447
display nearly equipotent saluretic activities in rats and dogs,
their relative antihypertensive effects are markedly different.
Hence, as noted earlier, the pronounced antihypertensive properties of MK-447 served to distinguish it from a subseries of
potent salidiuretic agents which emerged from this study. It is
interesting to note that the initial saluretic screening lead
(Ia) is not antihypertensive in the SH rat, whereas, the parent
structure, salicylamine (Compound VIa), has demonstrable, albeit
weak, antihypertensive activity in the SH rat, but it is devoid
of saluretic activity.

The third pharmacological attribute of MK-447, antiinflammatory activity, was demonstrated by its effect in reducing both
carrageenan-induced foot edema in rats and croton-oil induced
swelling in mouse ears ($\underline{12}$, $\underline{13}$). This action was suggested to
arise from the ability of MK-447 to scavenge an oxygen centered
free-radical released in the conversion of PGG_2 to PGH_2. Evidence has been provided to show that this radical is an important
inflammatory mediator ($\underline{12}$, $\underline{13}$).

The initial clinical study ($\underline{15}$) in normal volunteers has
shown that MK-447 is a potent, high-ceiling diuretic in man as
indicated by the natriuretic and kaliuretic data presented in
Figure 9. In this study, MK-447 displayed marked dose-related
saliuresis and diuresis with minimal kaliuresis. Recently, MK-447
was shown to elicit antihypertensive activity at diuretic doses
in man ($\underline{16}$). MK-447 is presently undergoing further clinical
investigation. Whether the adjunctive antiinflammatory activity
demonstrated for MK-447 in experimental animals will be observed
in man is yet to be established.

Acknowledgments - We are indebted to Ms. S. J. deSolms,
Mr. A. A. Deana and Mr. N. P. Gould for expert synthetic
assistance, to Mr. E. L. Cresson for the UV studies, to Dr. L.
S. Watson (deceased) and to Mr. H. F. Russo for the salidiuretic

TABLE XV. Relative Saluretic and Antihypertensive Activity

Compd.	Structure	Saluretic Score		Antihypertensive Score[a]	
		Rat	Dog	SH Rat	RH Dog
Ia		3	4	0	
VIa		0	0	1	
IXg		5	5	0	
IXi		5	5	1	1
VIIi		6	5	1	2
VIIk		6	5	2	2
MK–447		6	5	3	3

[a] Relative scores: outstanding activity = 3; moderate activity = 2; weak activity = 1; inactive = 0.

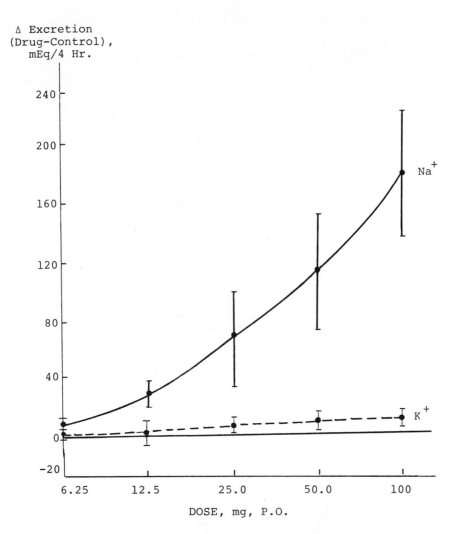

Figure 9. The natriuretic and kaliuretic effects of orally-administered MK-447 in normal human volunteers over a four-hr period. The data points are average values (Δ excretion = drug control) determined per volunteer in eight volunteers at each dose. Derived from the data of Affrime, M. B., et al. (15).

evaluations, to Dr. A. Scriabine and to Mr. C. T. Ludden for the
antihypertensive studies and to Dr. C. G. Van Arman for the
antiinflammatory results. Gratitude is expressed to Dr. J. L.
Humes for providing Figure 8, to Dr. K. Hoogsteen, Dr. J.
Springer and Mr. J. Hirschfield for the X-ray crystallographic
analysis of MK-447 free base and to Dr. G. M. Smith for the
CNDO/2 modeling studies. We wish to express our appreciation to
Drs. D. J. Tocco and J. E. Baer and their colleagues for the
metabolism studies, to Dr. R. O. Davies, Dr. J. M. Schrogie, Dr.
K. E. Tempero and Dr. B. Lei for the clinical investigations and
to Dr. J. M. Sprague (retired), Dr. C. A. Stone and Dr. R. F.
Hirschmann for their guidance and encouragement throughout the
course of this investigation.

<h2 style="text-align:center">Literature Cited and Notes</h2>

1. A series of manuscripts describing the details of this
investigation is in preparation by Stokker, G. E., Schultz,
E. M., Deana, A. A., deSolms, S. J., Sprague, J. M., Smith,
R. L. and Cragoe, E. J., Jr., for submission to J. Med. Chem.
2. Meadow, J., Berger, J. and Schert, R., Chim. Therap.
(1968), 3, 253.
3. Geschickter, C. and Meadow, J., U.S. Patent 3,080,365
(1968).
4. For an extensive review of the Tscherniac-Einhorn reaction,
see Zaugg, H. E. and Martin, W. B. in "Organic Reactions",
14, Adams, R., Blatt, A. H., Boekelheide, V., Cairns, T. L.,
Cope, A. C. and Niemann, C., Eds., J. Wiley and Sons, New York,
N. Y., 1965, pp 52-269.
5. Cragoe, E. J., Jr. and Schultz, E. M., U.S. Patent 4,029,816
(1977).
6. Since the Merck Molecular Modeling CNDO/2 program was
not parameterized for third and fourth row elements at the
time of this study, 6-chloro analog VIIi was subjected to
conformational analysis by the CNDO/2 calculational technique;
Smith, G. W., unpublished results.
7. Johnson, C. K., ORTEP, Rep. ORNL-3894 (1965), Oak Ridge
National Laboratory, Oak Ridge, Tenn.
8. Dietrich, S. W., Jorgensen, S. W., Kollman, P. A. and
Rothenberg, S., J. Am. Chem. Soc. (1976), 98, 8310.
9. Gregory, A. R. and Paddon-Row, M. W., J. Am. Chem. Soc.
(1976), 98, 7521.
10. Tocco, D. J., Walker, R. W., Arison, B. H., VandenHeuvel,
W. J. A., Stokker, G. E. and Smith, R. L., for submission
to Drug Dispos. Metab.
11. Scriabine, A., Watson, L. S., Russo, H. F., Ludden, C.
T., Sweet, C. S., Fanelli, G. M., Jr., Bohidar, N. and Stone,
C. A., Fed. Proc. (1978), 37, 921.
12. Kuehl, F. A., Jr., Humes, J. L., Egan, R. W., Ham, E.
A., Beveridge, G. C. and Van Arman, C. G., Nature (1977),
265, 170.
13. Kuehl, F. A., Jr., Egan, R. W., Humes, J. L., Beveridge,

G. C. and Van Arman, C. G., in "New Biochemical Aspects of
Prostaglandins and Thromboxanes", Fried, J. and Kharasch,
N., Eds., Academic Press, New York, N. Y., 1978.
14. Kuehl, F. A., Jr., Oien, H. G. and Ham, E. A. in "Prostaglandins in Cardiovascular and Renal Function", A. Scriabine,
F. A. Kuehl, Jr. and A. M. Lefer, Eds., Spectrum Publications,
New York, 1978, in press.
15. Affrime, M. B., Lowenthal, D. T., Onesti, G., Busby,
P., Schwartz, C. and Lei, B., Clin. Pharmacol. Ther. (1977),
21, 97.
16. Davies, R. O., personal communication (to be published).

RECEIVED August 21, 1978.

1-Aralkyl-2-pyrazolin-5-ones: A New Class of Highly Potent Diuretics with High Ceiling Activity

H. HORSTMANN, E. MÖLLER, E. WEHINGER, and K. MENG

Bayer Pharma Research Center, Postfach 10 17 09, D-56 Wuppertal 1, Federal Republic of Germany

The diuretics in use at the present time may be divided pharmacologically and clinically into compounds with either low-ceiling or high-ceiling activity.

Compounds having a low-ceiling activity exhibit a leveling-off or plateau in their diuretic action. Beyond a certain point, the diuretic effect is not increased by an increase in dosage. Typical low ceiling diuretics are the thiazides. Also, such compounds as chlorthalidone and mefruside belong to this group. A further characteristic of this group is the protracted duration of activity which is particularly advantageous in long-term treatment (Figure 1).

In contrast to this, the dose/activity curves of high-ceiling diuretics run almost linearly over a wide range. Such diuretics have a reserve in capacity and can, therefore, also be used on thiazide-resistant patients. A major disadvantage is their short duration of activity which is coupled with rebound phenomena. Representative compounds having this type of activity are ethacrynic acid, furosemide and bumetanide.

The medically most desirable combination of high-ceiling activity and protracted duration could not be realized until now. This was, therefore, the target of our own work in this area.

While it seemed improbable that progress could be made in this direction merely by working on known diuretics, we concentrated our attention on new classes of active substances.

Structural elements such as 1 and 2 which appear frequently in diuretic purines, triazines, pteridines, pyrazines and

pyrimidines, served as guidelines for selection.

A number of new diuretics, such as furosemide, bumetanide and triflocin (1), have amphoteric properties, so we also looked closely at compounds having acidic and basic functions in the same molecule.

As a result of this extensive search, we discovered a new class of agents represented by compound 3 a few years ago which possessed moderate diuretic activity in rats and dogs.

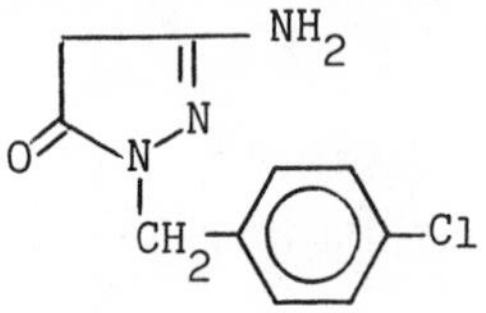

3

As may be seen, this is a 3-aminopyrazolin-5-one which is substituted in the 1-position by an aralkyl residue.

In contrast to the well-known and thoroughly investigated 3-amino-1-arylpyrazolin-5-ones, 3-amino-1-aralkylpyrazolin-5-ones had only been described in a few instances in the patent literature at the start of our work, and then, only as coupling components for magenta dyestuffs (2). The chemistry of this class will therefore be discussed first.

The preparation of 3-aminopyrazolin-5-ones (Formula 5) bearing aromatic substituents in the 1-position has been studied extensively by Weissberger and co-workers (3, 4, 5) and is carried out by reaction of arylhydrazines with cyanoacetate (Compound 4) in the presence of alkoxide. Certain heterocyclic hydrazine derivatives, such as 2-pyridylhydrazine, yield the isomeric 3-hydroxypyrazolin-5-imines (Formula 6) under these conditions.

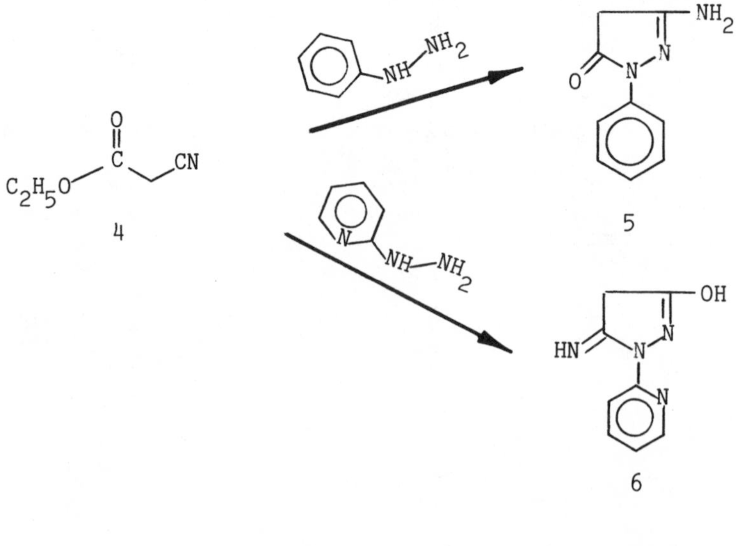

4

5

6

If β-amino-β-ethoxyacrylate (Compound 7) is employed instead of compound 4, then the 3-aminopyrazolin-5-one analogous to compound 5 is formed in both cases. In contrast to this behavior, aliphatic hydrazines, such as methylhydrazine (Compound 8), react even with compound 7 to give a mixture of 3-aminopyrazolin-5-one (Compound 9) and 3-hydroxypyrazolin-5-imine (Compound 10).

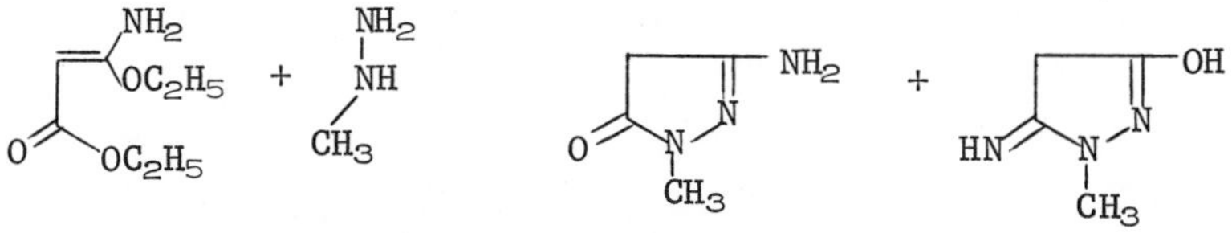

7   8   9   10

This result shows that both N-atoms of compound 8 are capable of reacting either with the ester function or with the imidate function of compound 7. One would expect a similar behavior from aralkylhydrazines. If one reacts 4-chlorobenzylhydrazine (Compound 11) with compound 7 under mild conditions for a short time and traps the primary product (Compound 12) with 4-nitrobenzaldehyde, then one isolates the hydrazone (Compound 13) in good yield.

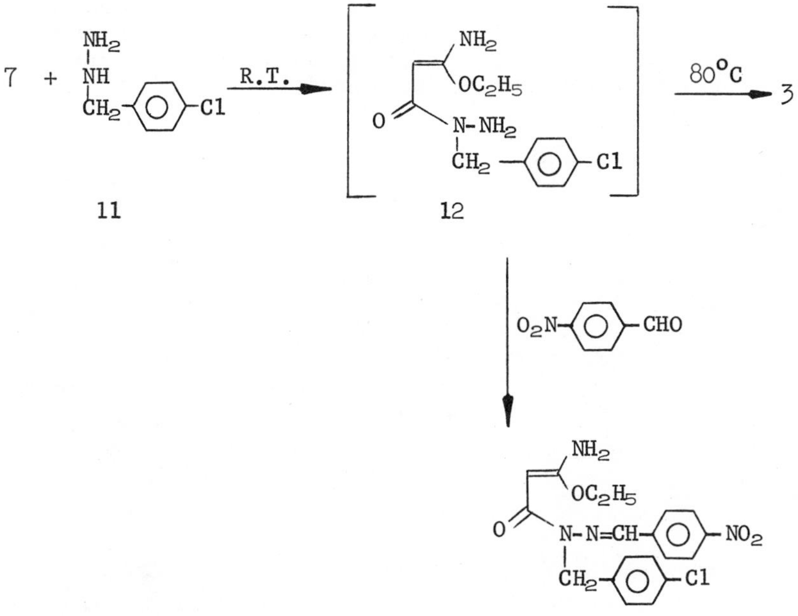

11   12

13

Under forcing conditions, compound 7 and compound 11 react
smoothly to give compound 3 in good yield. This shows that the
ester function reacts primarily and that the favored point of
attack is the substituted N-atom of compound 11.

If the imidate function is activated by salt formation, then
the amidrazone (Compound 14) is formed primarily, which does not
react with aldehydes. In this case, the unsubstituted N-atom of
compound 11 is the favored point of attack.

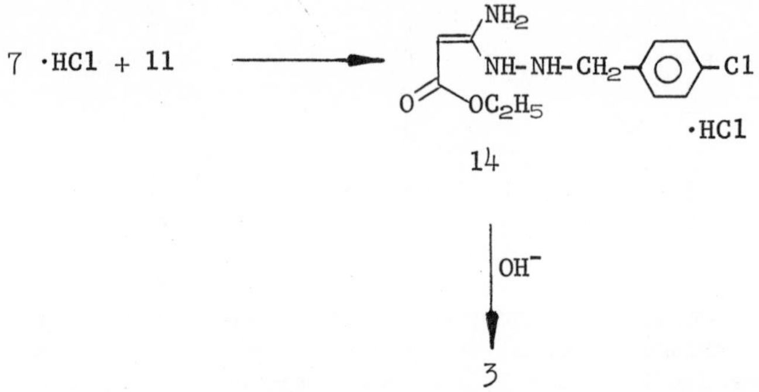

On addition of alkoxide, compound 14 is cyclized spontaneously to
compound 3 so that the same product results from both reactions.

If aralkylhydrazines are reacted directly with compound 4 in
the presence of alkoxide, then mixtures of the isomeric pyrazo-
lines (Compounds 16 and 17) are formed, as shown in the reaction
of 3,4-dichlorobenzylhydrazine (Compound 15).

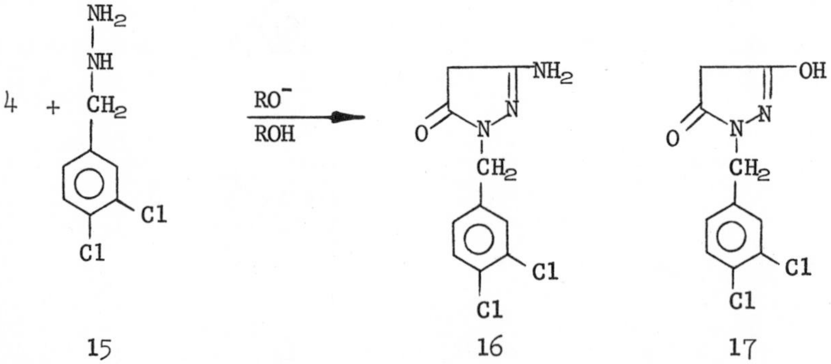

Since compound 3 is a polyfunctional species, it offers
countless opportunities for molecular variation; therefore, a
representative selection of analogs will be made for discussing
the effect of structural changes on diuretic activity. The
general formula 18 serves as a basis for this discussion.

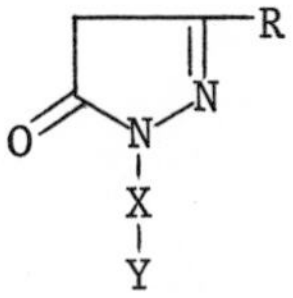

18

In Table I, the qualitative relationship is presented between structure and activity for the pyrazolin-5-ones (Structure 19) as a function of the substitution in the 3-position.

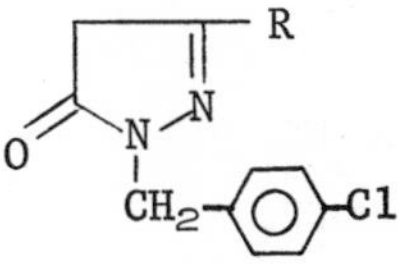

19

The results show that alkylation or acylation of the amino group causes a drastic loss of activity. Replacement of amino by a hydroxy- or carbonyl group or groups derived from these moieties also leads to weak or inactive compounds. In this regard, it was all the more surprising that compound 26 (and similar pyrazolin-5-ones substituted by lower alkyl groups) possessed a noteworthy diuretic potency. A plausible explanation for these results is not possible at the present time.
    The carbonyl group in the 5-position is of crucial impor-tance for activity. Inter alia, this may be seen by the fact that 1-(4-chlorobenzyl)-3-hydroxypyrazolin-5-imine, isomeric with Compound 3, and the corresponding 3,4-dichlorobenzyl derivative (Compound 15) have no diuretic activity. Furthermore, 3-amino-1-(4-chlorobenzyl)pyrazolin-5-imine, prepared from 4-chloro-benzylhydrazine and malonitrile, is also inactive.
    3-Aminopyrazolin-5-ones (Structure 32) possess amphoteric properties. It has been shown by NMR-studies that the equilib-rium Compound 32 ⇌ Compound 33 lies in favor of the enol form (Compound 33) in polar solvents.

TABLE I

The Qualitative Relationship between Structure and Activity
for the Pyrazolin-5-ones (Structure 19) with Variations (R)
in the 3-position.

No.	R	Activity
3	$-NH_2$	+
20	$-NHCH_3$	−
21	$-NHC_6H_5$	−
22	$-NH-COCH_3$	−
23	$-NH-CO-NHCH_3$	−
24	$-OH$	−
25	$-OC_2H_5$	−
26	$-CH_3$	+
27	$-C_6H_5$	−
28	$-COOC_2H_5$	−
29	$-COOH$	−
30	$-CONH_2$	−
31	$-CONHC-NH_2$ $\overset{\parallel}{NH}$	−

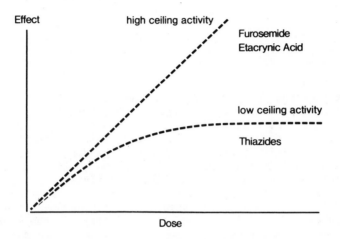

Figure 1.   Dose–effect curves of diuretics with high-ceiling and low-ceiling activity

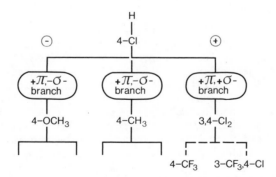

Figure 2.   Topliss-operation scheme greatly simplified

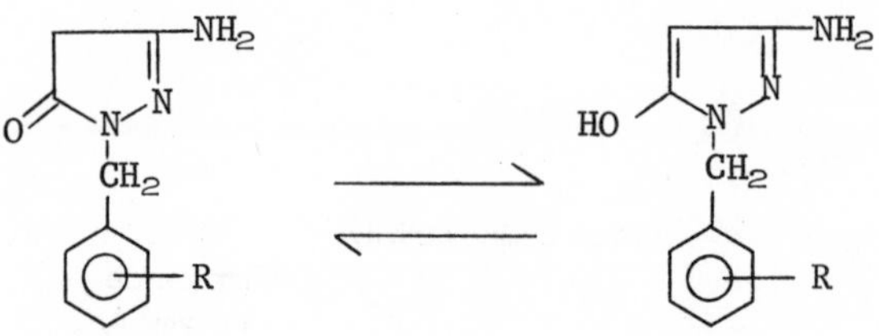

Our current data indicate that the capability of the compounds to undergo enolization seems to be of critical importance for activity. Inter alia, this also may be concluded from the fact that 3-aminopyrazolin-5-ones monoalkylated in the 4-position have diuretic activity, whereas, the analogs dialkylated in the 4-position are inactive. Replacement of the enolic hydroxyl group by a chlorine atom also leads to loss of activity.

The substitution pattern in the aromatic residue has been extensively investigated. In these studies, the operation scheme developed by Topliss (6) yielded good results. By the application of a somewhat simplified "Topliss tree" (Figure 2) to different subgroups of pyrazoles, we found that one always approached the area of optimal activity by following the $+\pi$, $+\delta$-branch as far as the 3,4-dichloro derivative.

Figure 3 shows the connection between the natural logarithm of the sodium excretion in the dog after oral administration of 3 mg/kg of each substance and the lipophilicity in the series of 3-amino-1-benzylpyrazolin-5-ones. The R_M value serves here as a measure of the lipophilicity (Figure 3). If one takes into account that these data were orientating values obtained on the intact animal, i.e., two dogs per substance, then the result, with a correlation coefficient of 0.63 and a random sample size of 24, may be regarded as satisfactory and serve as an aid for planning new syntheses. The results would be better if the pharmacological data could be refined by multiple repetition. This was only possible with a small number of compounds due to limited capacity.

We obtained very interesting results by variation of the bridge X between the heterocyclic and aryl moieties. A selection of compounds of general formula 34, which serves to illustrate this, is contained in Table II.

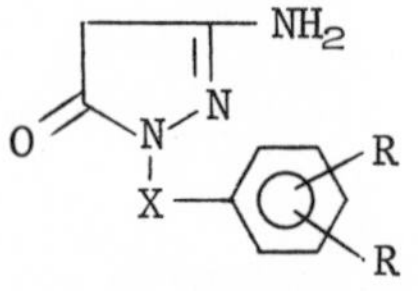

R=H, CH$_3$, Cl

34

TABLE II

The Average Activities of Compounds on Variation
of the Bridge X between Heterocycle
and Aryl Residue (Formula 34).

Subgroup	X	Activity *
I	-	-
II	$-CH_2-$	+
III	$-CH(CH_3)-$	+++
IV	$-CH_2-CH_2-$	+
V	$-CH_2-CH_2-O-$	++
VI	$-CH_2-CH=CH-$	++
VII	$-CH_2-CH_2-CH_2-$	-

*dog, 3 mg/kg p.o.;

-	<500 µEq	Na^+/Kg
+	500–1000	"
++	1000–2000	"
+++	>2000	"

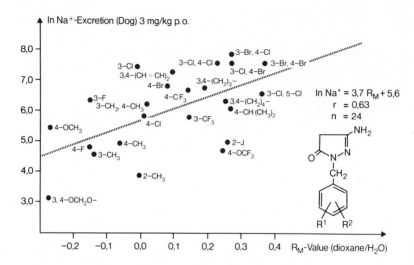

Figure 3. *Quantitative structure activity relationship between sodium excretion in the dog and lipophilicity*

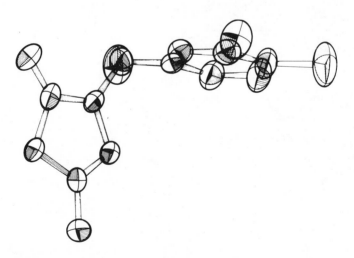

Figure 4. *X-ray crystal structure of muzolimine*

The results should, however, only indicate a trend in activity
which was observed in the dog by variation of the bridge X.
(Within the individual subgroups, the average was taken of the
results obtained on compounds with different substitution patterns.)

An important guideline for continued work in this class of
compounds was the observation that 3-amino-1-arylpyrazolin-5-ones
(Subgroup I) were inactive; 3-amino-1-benzylpyrazolin-5-ones with
a methyl branching in the methylene group (Subgroup III) were
highly active. This is illustrated by the comparison of some
unbranched 3-amino-1-benzylpyrazolin-5-ones with the corresponding
branched derivatives (Table III, General Formula 35).

35

From the several hundred pyrazolin-5-ones synthesized in
these laboratories, muzolimine (BAY g 2821, Compound 38, 3-amino-
1-(3,4-dichloro-α-methylbenzyl)pyrazolin-5-one) was selected for
clinical trials.

38

Figure 4 shows the X-ray crystal structure of muzolimine. In Table
IV, some physicochemical data for muzolimine and furosemide are
listed. These data show that BAY g 2821 is noticeably more
lipophilic than furosemide, which is probably of great significance in explaining their different pharmacokinetics.

In Figure 5, the dose/activity curve in the dog is shown for
different electrolytes. As can be seen, doses of muzolimine in
the range 0.1 mg/kg to 3 mg/kg cause an almost linear increase in
the excretion rate of chloride and sodium ions. The potassium
excretion is only significantly increased by doses above 1 mg/kg.
The bicarbonate excretion remains almost unaffected. Thus, muzolimine behaves similar to furosemide and must be added to the group
of "high ceiling" diuretics.

An even clearer demarcation with respect to furosemide and
the special activity profile of BAY g 2821 is seen when one
studies the activity vs. time curve after a single dose of 1
mg/kg. When one measures the excretion volume and electrolyte

TABLE III

Comparison of the Activities of Some Unbranched
3-Amino-1-Benzylpyrazolin-5-Ones with the Activities
of the Corresponding Branched Derivatives (Formula 35).

No.	-X-	-Ar-	Activity*
3	$-CH_2-$	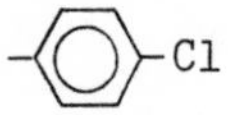 ⟨◯⟩-Cl	+
36	$-CH(CH_3)-$	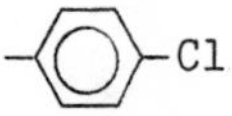 ⟨◯⟩-Cl	+++
37	$-CH_2-$	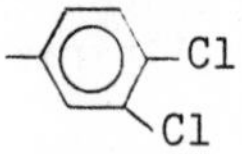 ⟨◯⟩-Cl, Cl	++++
38	$-CH(CH_3)-$	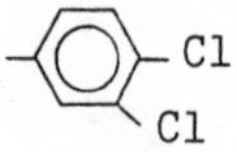 ⟨◯⟩-Cl, Cl	++++++ (muzolimine)
39	$-CH_2-$	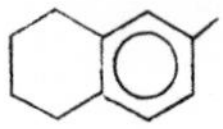 ◯◯	+
40	$-CH(CH_3)-$	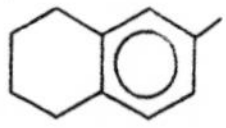 ◯◯	++++

*Increased sodium excretion; dog, 3 mg/kg p.o./1 hr.

+ = 500 $\pm$ 100 µEq Na^+/Kg

TABLE IV

Physicochemical Properties of Muzolimine
in Comparison with Furosemide

	Furosemide	Muzolimine
pK_a	3.9	9.2
lg P (octanol/H_2O)	-.83	2.29
R_M (ethanol/H_2O)	-.62	-.84
R_M (dioxane/H_2O)	-.67	-.33

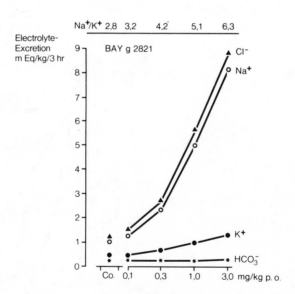

*Figure 5.   Dose–activity curves in the dog after appli-
cation of muzolimine*

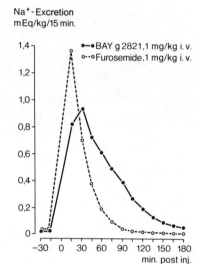

Figure 6. Time–response curves in the dog without substitution after a single dose of 1 mg/kg

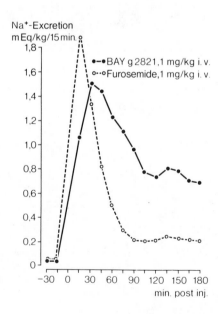

Figure 7. Time–response curves in the dog with substitution after a single dose of 1 mg/kg

quantities at short intervals over 180 minutes, it is found that
the action of furosemide is of rapid onset but soon drops away,
whereas, with muzolimine, the initial increase in action is
slower, but the duration is longer (Figure 6).

These differences become even more distinct when the salt
and volume losses caused by the substance are replaced by an
infusion carefully matched to the excretion rate. By this means,
the counter-regulation effect in the healthy animal is nullified
and the salt and water reserves present in the edematous patient
are simulated. Under these conditions, one can see that the
activity of BAY g 2821 is not only of distinctly longer duration,
but is also higher than that of furosemide with respect to the
total excretion (Figure 7).

For approximately two years, muzolimine has been under
clinical test. A whole series of carefully controlled studies
have been completed in the meantime and some have been published
(7-13). In these studies, the activity of muzolimine, especially
the novel combination of high-ceiling and long-acting activities
on different forms of edema, particularly on cardiac and hepato-
genic edemas, has been confirmed.

Literature Cited

1. Meng, K. and Loew, D., "Diuretika: Chemie, Pharmakologie,
Therapie," 232, Georg Thieme Verlag, Stuttgart (1974).
2. Vanden Eynde, H. A., Pollet, R. J. and DeCat, A. H., U.S.
Patent 3,563,745 (1971).
3. Weissberger, A. and Porter, H. D., J. Amer. Chem. Soc. (1942),
64, 2133.
4. Weissberger, A., Porter, H. D. and Gregory, W. A., J. Amer.
Chem. Soc. (1944), 66, 1851.
5. Graham, B., Porter H. D. and Weissberger, A., J. Amer.
Chem. Soc. (1949), 71, 983.
6. Topliss, J. G., J. Med. Chem. (1972), 15, 1006.
7. Möller, E., Horstmann, H., Meng, K. and Loew, D., Experientia
(1977), 33, 382.
8. Berg, K. J., Jorstad, S. and Tromsdal, A., Pharmatherapeutica
(1976), 1, 319.
9. Fauchald, P. and Lind, E., Pharmatherapeutica (1977), 1,
409.
10. Hoppeseyler, G., Heissler, A., Coppencastrop, M., Schindler,
M. Schollmeyer, P. and Ritter, W., Pharmatherapeutica (1977),
1, 422.
11. Loew, D., Curr. Med. Res. Opin. (1977), 4, 455.
12. Loew, D. and Meng, K., Pharmatherapeutica (1977), 1, 333.
13. Loew, D. and Meng, K., Naunyn-Schmiedeberg's Arch. Pharmacol.
(1977), 297, (Suppl. 2), R38.

RECEIVED August 21, 1978.

9

Quincarbate: A Representative of a New Class of Diuretics with 1,4-Dioxino[2,3-g]quinolone Structure

TH. A. C. BOSCHMAN, J. VAN DIJK', J. HARTOG, and J. N. WALOP

Philips–Duphar B.V., Research Laboratories, 1380 AA, Weesp, The Netherlands

During an investigation of new quinolone derivatives (Figure 1), which were synthesized mainly for anticoccidiosis testing, it was found that some of these compounds possessed potent diuretic activity (1).

In this paper, we will discuss, in turn: (a) the structure-activity relationships (SAR) of the compounds of the series, (b) the physicochemical properties of some representative compounds, (c) the pharmacological profile and the metabolism of quincarbate, the compound selected for human pharmacological investigation and (d) the preliminary results of the evaluation of quincarbate in humans.

STRUCTURE-ACTIVITY RELATIONSHIPS

The diuretic activity was determined in saline loaded rats after oral administration of the compounds according to a modification of the method of Lipschitz (2). The volume of excreted urine as well as its electrolyte contents were measured over a 5-hour period. The activity was expressed as an ED_{200} value, i.e., the dose (mg/kg) which gave a 100% increase in the urinary volume over the control value.

Compound 1 (Figure 2) is a prototype structure which possesses the characteristics essential for diuretic activity. Variation of the ring structure, as well as, of the location of the substituents generally led to compounds with no oral activity at 50 mg/kg (Figure 3). Reorientation of the $EtOCH_2$-group to the vicinal carbon atom in the dioxino ring, as in compound 2, or the reorientation of the carboxyl group in the pyridone ring, as in compound 3, produced a considerable decrease in activity or to inactive compounds. Contraction (Compound 4), expansion (Compound 5), or opening (Compound 6), or reorientation (Compound 7) of the dioxino ring also produced inactive compounds. Likewise, the presence of methyl groups on the pyridone nucleus had a disastrous effect on the activity (Compounds 8 and 9).

Variation of R_3 revealed that a small alkoxyalkyl substituent

' Address correspondence to this author.

0-8412-0464-0/78/47-083-**140**$05.00/0
© American Chemical Society

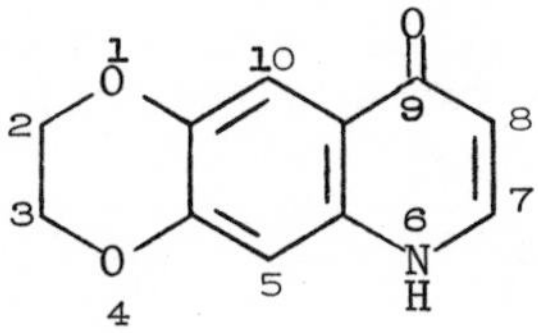

Figure 1. 1,4-Dioxino[2,3-g]-quinolone

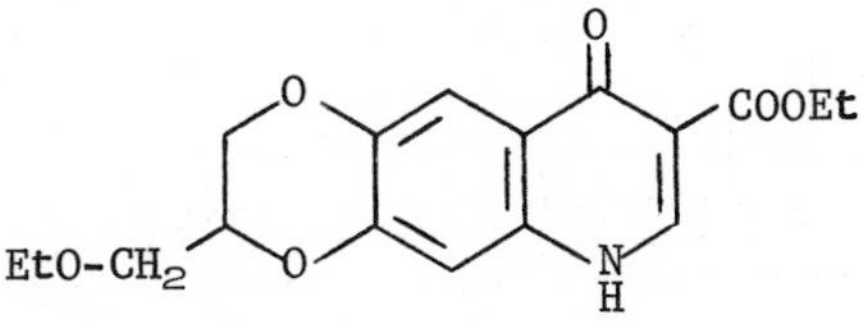

Figure 2. Compound 1, a prototype of the series

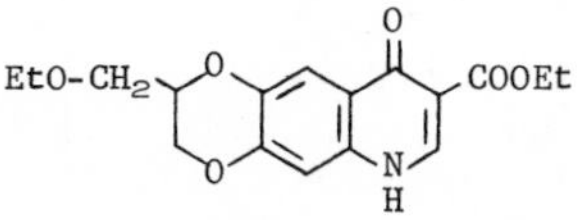

2

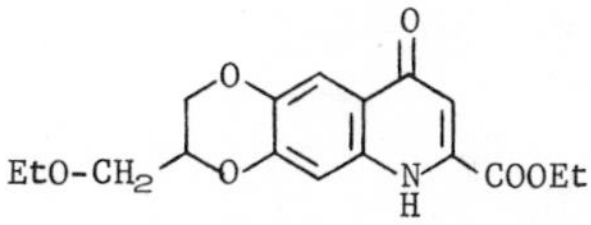

3

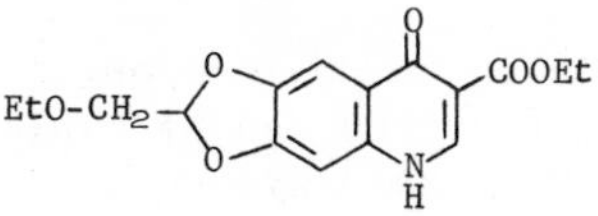

4

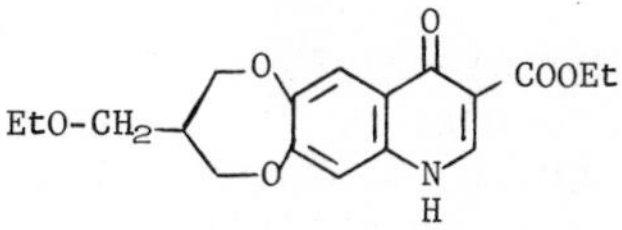

5

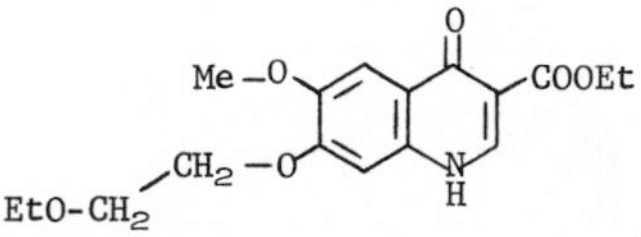

6

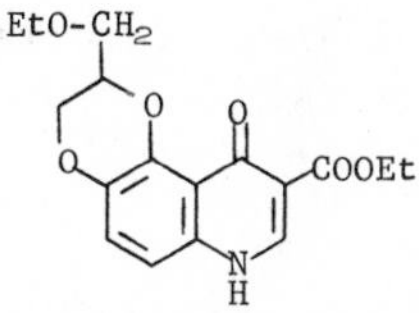

7

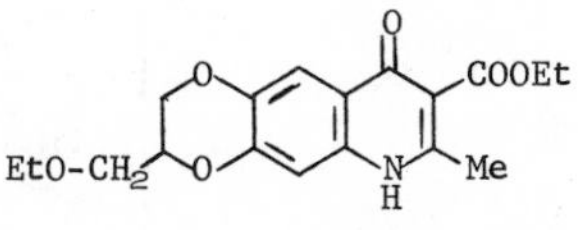

8

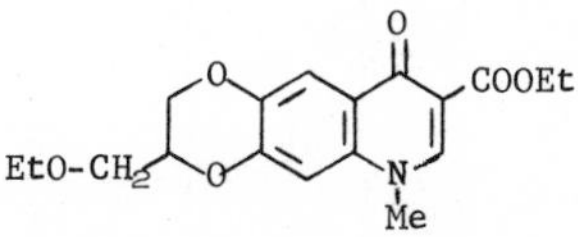

9

Figure 3. Inactive (a, b) analogs in which substituents or rings have been rearranged.

(a) Diureses estimated in saline-loaded rats; (b) inactive means: no activity at 50 mg/kg, orally.

was essential, since compounds 15, 16, 17, 18 and 19 were inactive, and it also showed that the oxymethylene bridge appeared
optimal (Table I).

Table I.   Effect of variation of R_3 in

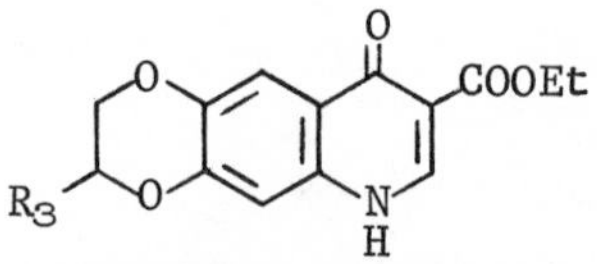

no.	R_3	ED_{200}		no.	R_3	ED_{200} (mg/kg)
1	EtO-CH$_2$	3.8		15	H	
10	HO-CH$_2$-	10		16	Me-	>50 or
11	MeO-CH$_2$-	10		17	Cl-CH$_2$-	inactive compounds
12	PrO-CH$_2$-	15		18	MeO-CO-	
13	MeO-CH$_2$-CH$_2$-O-CH$_2$-	4		19	n-C$_8$H$_{17}$-O-CH$_2$-	
14	EtO-CH$_2$-CH$_2$-	~ 20				

The substituent R_8 (Table II) seemed to be less critical,
since the carboxy or ethoxy carbonyl function can be replaced by
an acetyl group (Compound 21) or even by an alkyl group (Compound
24).   Whether the activities of these various compounds are due to
metabolism has not been established.

Table II.   Effect of variation of R_8 in

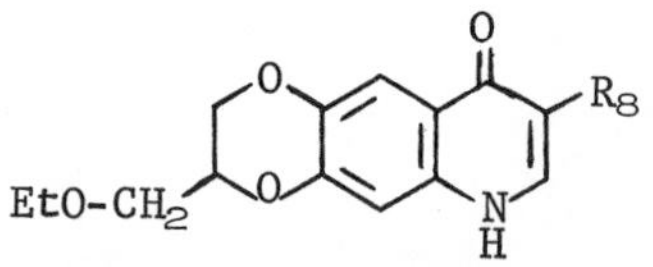

no.	R_8	ED_{200}		no.	R_8	ED_{200} (mg/kg)
1	-COOEt	3.8		25	-CO-NH$_2$	
20	-COOH	7		26	-C≡N	
21	-CO-Me	12		27	-CH$_2$-NH$_2$	>50
22	-CH$_2$-OH	4		28	-H	or inactive
23	-CHOH-Me	11		29	-Br	compounds
24	-Et	10		30	-NH$_2$	
				31	-NO$_2$	

Substitution of the benzene nucleus produced marked change (Table III) in diuretic activity.

Table III. Effect of variation of R_5 and R_{10} in

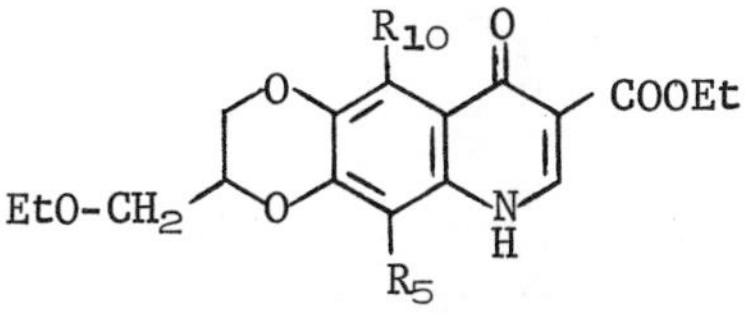

no.	$R_{10}(R_5=H)$	ED_{200}	no.	R_{10}	R_5	ED_{200} (mg/kg)
1	H	3.8	38	NH_2	H	50
32	Me	4	39	OMe	H	
33	Cl	0.08	40	H	Cl	>50
34	Br	∿0.4	41	Cl	Cl	or
35	CF_3	∿0.5				inactive
36	NO_2	∿3				compounds
37	NHAc	13				

When R_{10} was a lipophilic, electronegative group, as in compounds 33, 34, 35 and 36, activity was increased, especially when R_{10}=Cl, as in compound 33. Compound 33 (whose recommended INN name is quincarbate) was the most active member of the series. Electron donating groups for R_{10}, e.g., NH_2 (Compound 38) and OMe (Compound 39), produced a considerable decrease in activity. It is remarkable that when the other hydrogen atom (R_5) was substituted by Cl, as in compounds 40 and 41, activity was totally lost.

Some variants of R_9 induce the pyridone ring I to assume its tautomeric form II (Figure 4). If R_9 is an oxygen atom, the pyridone configuration I dominated almost completely, as confirmed by IR data. This was also the case with compound 43 and probably with compound 42, but if R_9=OMe (Compound 44) or Cl (Compound 46), only tautomer II is possible. Since among the compounds which exist in one or the other tautomeric form, both active as well as inactive compounds are found (Table IV), the actual ring structure would appear not to be relevant.

Table IV.   Effect of variation of $R_\ominus$ in

no.	$R_\ominus$	ED_{200}		no.	$R_\ominus$		ED_{200} (mg/kg)
1	OH	3.8		45	NHPr	⎫	> 50
42	SH	~ 13		46	Cl	⎬	or
43	NH_2	~ 13				⎭	inactive
44	OMe	30					compounds

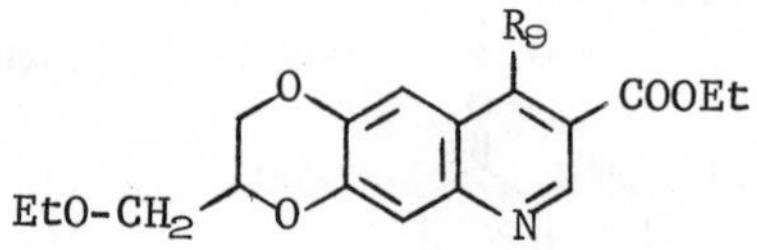

The SAR may be summarized by the statement that the tricyclic compound must be linear and unsubstituted at positions 2, 5, 6 and 7. Substitution at position 3 with a hydroxymethyl or alkoxymethyl group is necessary, while at position 8, a substituent such as a carboxyl, alkoxycarbonyl, hydroxyalkyl, acetyl, or alkyl group must be present. The oxygen atom normally present at position 9 may be replaced by certain groups, and substitution at position 10 by lipophilic electronegative groups increases the activity. A QSAR for substituents at position 10 confirmed these statements. In the calculations concerning R_8, three deviations from the regression were found, i.e., with compounds 28, 29 and 31.

PHYSICOCHEMICAL PROPERTIES

The compounds of this series possess an extremely low solubility in water (Table V). The partition coefficients indicated a rather lipophilic character, but the solubility in lipophilic solvents was generally very low, being far less than 0.1% in most solvents. The ester, quincarbate (Compound 33), exhibits good solubility (>10%) only in strongly protonating solvents, while the acids (Compounds 47 and 51) form soluble salts in aqueous alkali.

Table V. Comparison of solubility and partition coefficient with diuretic activity in rats

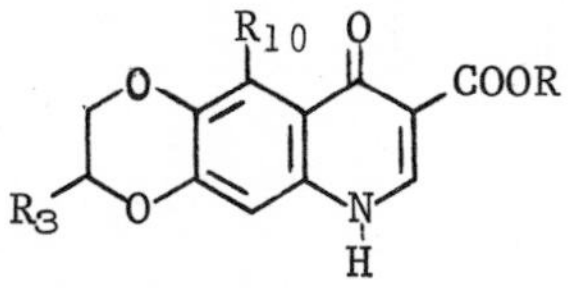 No.	R$_3$	R$_{10}$	R	Solubility in water at pH 6 at 20°C (mg/L)	Partition coefficient octanol/water at pH 7.5	Diuretic activity ED$_{200}$ (mg/kg)
1	EtOCH$_2$	H	Et	30	> 50	3.8
33	EtOCH$_2$	Cl	Et	1	> 50	0.08
47	EtOCH$_2$	Cl	H	0.5	25	0.14
48	EtOCH$_2$	Cl	CH$_2$-CH$_2$OH	10		0.2
49	EtOCH$_2$	Cl	CH$_2$-CHOH-CH$_2$OH	20	4.5	0.5
50	EtOCH$_2$	Cl	CH$_2$-O-COMe	1.6		1.0
51	HOCH$_2$	Cl	H	1.5	1.7	∼1
52	HOCH$_2$	Cl	Et	30	5.7	∼0.1

Since the extremely low solubility (<30 mg/L) of the compounds might influence the bioavailability, some compounds were synthesized with more hydrophilic substituents (Table V, Compounds 48, 49, 51 and 52). However, no improvement in activity was accomplished.

It may be concluded that, in spite of the role played by the lipophilic character of certain groups (e.g., Cl at R$_{10}$), the lipophilicity of the whole molecule (partition coefficient) does not seem to be an important factor in the level of activity that is achieved (compare compounds 33 and 47 with 52, and compound 1 with 33). Also, an extremely low solubility does not seem to have a negative effect on the activity in the rat.

PHARMACOLOGICAL PROFILE

Quincarbate (Compound 33, Figure 5) was selected for development as a possible drug for human therapy. The various existing diuretics can be divided into two classes: "high ceiling" diuretics, of which furosemide is a well-known representative, and "low ceiling" diuretics, a class to which most diuretics of the thiazide type belong. The difference can be demonstrated most clearly in saline-loaded rats using the Lipschitz method (2). Using this procedure, quincarbate was shown to be a "high ceiling" diuretic with an efficacy comparable to that of furosemide

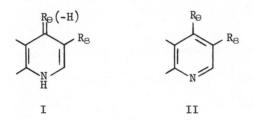

Figure 4. Tautomeric forms of the pyridine
moiety

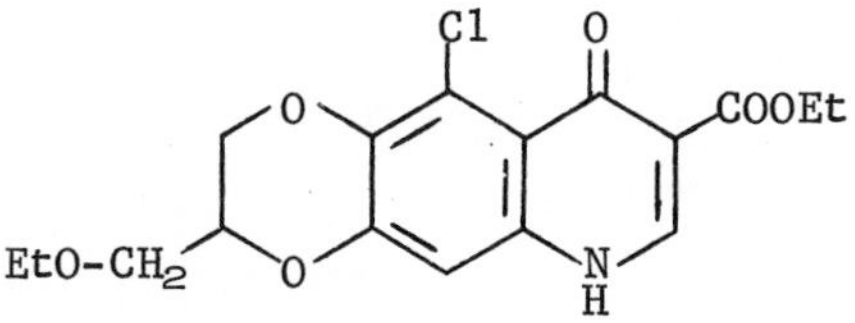

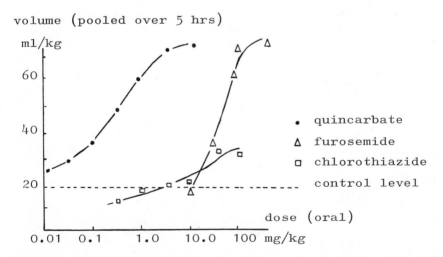

Figure 5. Structure of quincarbate

Figure 6. Dose–response relationships in male albino rats (strain Wistar-TNO, 160
± 20 g), six animals per dose group

(Figure 6). Significant diuretic effects of quincarbate in rats are elicited at doses which are at least 200 times lower than the minimum dose required for furosemide and chlorothiazide. However, since the dose/response curves do not run parallel, a strict comparison of the potencies is not possible.

The electrolyte excretion caused by quincarbate, furosemide and chlorothiazide, respectively, parallels their diuretic response (Figure 7). Over the complete dose range, quincarbate gives a more favorable ratio of the Na^+/K^+ excretion when compared to furosemide, and it is even better when compared to chloro-thiazide (Figure 8).

The dehydration of the animals caused by effective diuretics masks their effectiveness over longer time intervals. In order to prevent such an interference in the study of the duration of action, the rats were intermittently loaded with saline in a volume equal to the volume of urine excreted in the preceding period. From Figure 9, it is clear that quincarbate has a rapid onset of action, as does furosemide. However, the action continues over a period of seven hours, after which it gradually subsides, whereas furosemide has a much shorter duration of action.

When tested in rats not loaded with saline at a daily dose of 0.1 mg/kg for 14 days, the diuretic activity of quincarbate remained undiminished. No rebound effects were observed after discontinuing the administration of the drug. Also, in water-deprived rats, a diuretic effect was clearly seen.

Quincarbate shows a remarkable variation in its diuretic effectiveness in various species. In dogs, an ED_{200} value of 5 mg/kg orally was obtained. It is noteworthy that in this species the natriuretic response was more pronounced than the diuretic response (Figure 10). Surprisingly, in mice an antidiuretic effect was noted at low doses (1 mg/kg), whereas, at higher doses (46 and 100 mg/kg), some diuretic effect was apparent. In hamsters, quincarbate exhibited only marginal activity.

From both in vitro and in vivo studies, it can be concluded that quincarbate is not a carbonic anhydrase inhibitor. It exerted its diuretic effect even in drug-induced acidotic rats. The potency was unaffected in adrenalectomized rats; furthermore, no direct aldosterone antagonism was observed. In rats with artificially induced edema (partial hepatectomy), quincarbate proved to be highly effective.

Quincarbate was tested for antihypertensive activity in spontaneously hypertensive (SH) rats (3). The drug was administered orally, followed 20 hours later by a second dose; then 4 hours later, the blood pressure was measured by a cannula in the caudal artery. A slight activity was observed at 1 mg/kg, and a maximum effect was seen at 5 mg/kg. A prolonged action was indicated by noting that the original blood pressure was somewhat decreased even 20 hours after the first dose. With a dose of 5 mg/kg, the actual lowering (in mm Hg) was from 169.0 $\pm$ 9.6 to

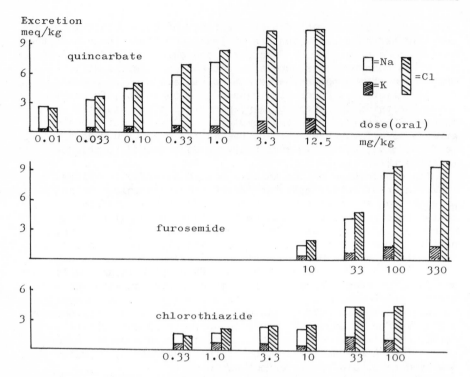

Figure 7.   Dose–response of electrolyte excretion in saline-loaded rats. Six animals per dose group were used. Determinations of electrolytes were performed in pooled urine samples excreted in the five-hour period.

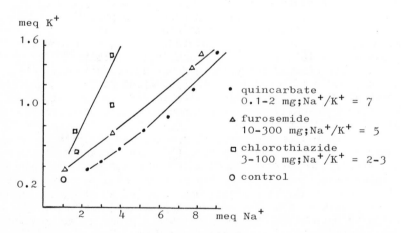

Figure 8.   Ratios of Na⁺:K⁺ excretion in saline-loaded rats. (Further details in legend of Figure 7.)

138.3 + 7.3 at the fourth hour on the second day (3). In renal
hypertensive rats, no conclusive effects were found with either
quincarbate or furosemide. Following oral administration of
quincarbate to rats at doses of up to 100 mg/kg, no toxic or
neurotoxic phenomena were observed. Also, in chronic toxicity
studies with rats and dogs, no serious side effects were observed
at doses of 50 mg/kg. In rabbits and rats, quincarbate did not
adversely affect pregnancy, nor did it show teratogenic potential.

METABOLISM

The metabolism of quincarbate was studied in rats, dogs,
monkeys and humans by means of ^{14}C-labelled material. From a
number of experiments in normal rats as well as in rats with
cannulated or ligated bile duct, it can be deduced that the ratio
of urinary to biliary excretion of metabolites of quincarbate is
2:1. The material that is excreted in the bile does not enter an
enterohepatic circulation but is excreted in the feces.

Using the above-mentioned ratio, we calculated the amount of
absorption on the basis of the urinary excretion of radioactive
material. In all species, the degree of absorption was strongly
dose dependent. In rats, the degree of absorption decreased from
45% at a dose of 1 mg/kg to 15% at the dose of 16 mg/kg. In dogs,
the absorption percentage declined from 40% at the dose of 0.1
mg/kg to 2.25% at 50 mg/kg. In monkeys, at a dose of 1 mg/kg, the
absorption was 10%. In humans, the degree of absorption declined
from 60% at 0.015 mg/kg to 55% at 0.075 mg/kg and finally to 44%
at 0.3 mg/kg. Hence, within the therapeutic range, about 50% of
the dose will be absorbed. Urinary excretion in all species ended
within 24 hours.

Plasma levels of radioactive material were extremely low at
all times in rats, dogs and humans. Maximum levels tended to be
reached within one to three hours. Neither unchanged quincarbate
nor the corresponding acid, nor even conjugates, were found in the
excretion products. In the urine of the rat and the monkey, seven
metabolites could be identified. In dogs and man, only three of
these were found. Of these three, the one which occurred in the
major proportion by far proved to be compound 51 (Figure 11).
Thus, both ether and ester hydrolysis must have occurred.

Since both the hydroxymethyl derivative of the acid, compound
51, as well as of the corresponding ester, compound 52, show high
activity (Table V), these products may also play an important role
in the observed diuretic effect.

Since one of the characteristics of quincarbate is its species
dependent diuretic activity, a study was conducted to reveal
whether or not this was a matter of metabolism. The diuretic
activity of compound 52, the ester of the main metabolite, was
studied in various species. In dogs, compound 52 showed an
activity comparable to that of quincarbate, and, in mice,
it was completely inactive at doses up to 10 mg/kg. Therefore,

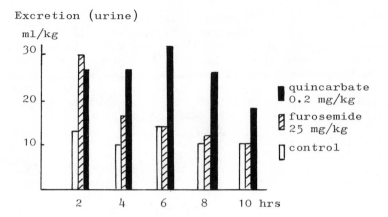

Figure 9.   Duration of diuretic action in rats after single oral administration. Six animals per group were used. Rats were intermittently
loaded with saline.

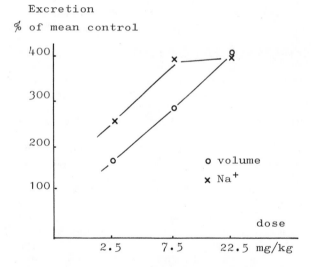

Figure 10.   Urine and Na⁺ excretion in beagle dogs after
oral administration of quincarbate. Seven dogs per dose
group were used. Excreted urine was pooled after seven
hours.

Figure 11.   Main excretion product of quincarbate and its ester. 51: R = H. 52: R =
Et.

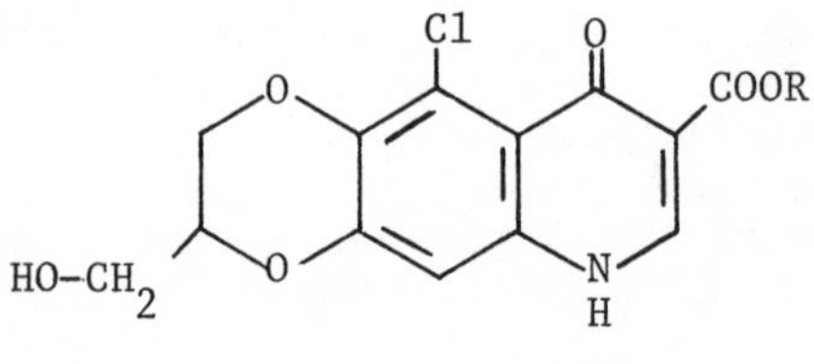

it is unlikely that the species dependence is due to different degrees of formation of the active metabolites. It is possible that the degree of absorption of quincarbate in the various species determines, to a certain extent, the variation in diuretic potency.

HUMAN PHARMACOLOGY

The effect of quincarbate on the excretion of urine and of urinary electrolytes has been investigated in six small studies (4-8), including 34 healthy volunteers. In all these studies, quincarbate was given as a single oral dose, but several subjects ingested the drug in different dosages on subsequent test days. This resulted in a total of 84 single-dose administrations at different dose levels. The following preliminary conclusions may be drawn:

Potency. In the range of 5 to 40 mg, the dose/response curve of quincarbate is very flat. This might be partially explained by incomplete absorption at the higher doses in man. Quincarbate proved to be quite potent; thus, 10 to 20 mg given orally showed natriuretic effects comparable with those of 100 mg hydrochlorothiazide (4) (Table VI).

Table VI.   Diuretic response in humans to quincarbate and hydrochlorothiazide (4) (double-blind study involving six healthy male volunteers between the ages of 22 and 32 years).

Mean Cumulative Response

	Diuresis (ml)		Natriuresis (meq)		Na^+/K^+ ratio	
	after 12 hrs	after 24 hrs	after 12 hrs	after 24 hrs	after 12 hrs	after 24 hrs
Placebo	695	1218	61	126	2.0	2.7
quincarbate						
5 mg	978	1598	145	239	3.4	4.0
10 mg	1162	1903	152	266	2.9	3.7
20 mg	1082	1998	170	309	3.4	4.1
40 mg	1315	2217	158	274	2.5	3.2
hydrochloro-thiazide						
100 mg	1223	2110	183	310	4.2	4.9

The oral activity of quincarbate was compared in four studies
(4-6, 8) with that of furosemide. While 5 (or 20) mg of quincarbate proved to be more natriuretic than 20-25 mg of furosemide,
40 mg of furosemide sometimes showed a lesser and sometimes a
greater effect than 20 mg of quincarbate. With 80 mg of furosemide, greater natriuresis and diuresis could be achieved than
with quincarbate. Table VII gives the results of one of these
studies.

Pattern of Activity. Quincarbate's diuretic activity starts
within one hour after its oral ingestion and lasts for at least
8-9 hours, but (as can be inferred from Table VI) diuresis and
natriuresis continue even during the 12-24 hour interval.

Table VII. Diuretic response in humans to quincarbate and
            furosemide (5) (double-blind placebo-controlled
            cross-over study involving four male and four
            female healthy volunteers between the ages of
            22 and 61 years).

	Mean cumulative response after 8 hrs		
	Diuresis (ml)	Natriuresis (meq)	Na^+/K^+ ratio
Placebo	608	40.8	2.0
quincarbate			
5 mg	1232	137.3	4.6
10 mg	1262	143.9	3.5
20 mg	1204	142.4	3.9
furosemide			
20 mg	1214	117.2	3.3
40 mg	1772	180.8	4.2

While there is an increase in urinary K^+ excretion, it is less
than the corresponding increase in urinary Na^+ excretion. This
results in a favorable Na^+/K^+ ratio, comparable to that following
ingestion of furosemide. Both the diuretic and natriuretic
response are also well maintained in dehydrated subjects.
    The main anion excreted concurrently with the increase in Na^+
and K^+ excretion is the chloride ion. There is no indication of
any inhibition of tubular bicarbonate reabsorption. Neither the
glomerular filtration rate (as measured by the rate of inulin
clearance) nor the renal plasma flow (as measured by the p-
aminohippuric acid clearance) are affected by quincarbate.

Side Effects and Tolerance. Up to the present time, quincarbate has been tolerated extremely well; no clinical side effects of any importance have been observed. Occasionally, a slight decrease in serum Na$^+$ and/or K$^+$ was noted, as might be expected with any potent diuretic.

CINICAL STUDIES

Our clinical studies to assess quincarbate's efficacy and side effects are in their early stages. Only one (6) small double-blind cross-over study in hospitalized patients with peripheral cardiac edema has been completed. In this study, considerable improvement of clinical edema was apparent in all patients. In the cross-over study, an oral dose of 10 mg quincarbate was compared with 50 mg hydrochlorothiazide; the overall response to both drugs (improvement of edema, loss of weight, excretion of urine and Na$^+$, favorable Na$^+$/K$^+$ ratio, excretion of other electrolytes) was quite similar.

CONCLUSIONS

(1) Some dioxino/2,3-g/quinoline derivatives exhibit extremely potent diuretic activity with a high ceiling character in the rat.

(2) The structures of this group differ markedly from those of established diuretics.

(3) The structural variations permissible for diuretic activity are very limited.

(4) The most active compound, quincarbate (Figure 5), which at an oral dose of 0.08 mg/kg doubled the volume of the urine excreted by the rat, was studied extensively.

(5) Upon repeated administration of quincarbate to rats, no tolerance or rebound effects were noted.

(6) The diuretic activity of quincarbate was species dependent; it exhibited potent activity in rats and humans, moderate activity in dogs and monkeys and only marginal activity in mice and hamsters.

(7) The main metabolite of quincarbate (compound 51) also possessed diuretic activity.

(8) In chronic toxicity studies in rats and dogs, no notable toxic effects were observed at oral doses up to 50 mg/kg.

(9) In healthy humans, an oral dose of 5 mg of quincarbate showed a marked diuretic and natriuretic effect; and yet, even at the highest dose used (20 mg), no side effects of any importance were noted.

(10) In patients with peripheral cardiac edema, a considerable improvement of the edema was apparent with low doses (10 mg orally). However, further studies will be required before quincarbate can be assigned its place among future therapeutics.

Acknowledgments - We acknowledge the efforts of all our colleagues in the research laboratories of Philips-Duphar who have

involved in the studies which we have described. We mention
especially K. S. Liem, M.D., who coordinated the studies in man,
Dr. J. B. v.d. Schoot, who carried out the metabolic studies, and
Mr. J. Tipker, who provided the valuable QSAR calculations.

Literature Cited

1. Dijk, J. van, Hartog, J. and Boschman, Th.A.C., J. Med. Chem.
(1976), 19, 982.
2. Lipschitz, W. L., Hadidian, Z. and Kerpscar, A., J. Pharmacol.
Exp. Ther. (1943), 92, 97.
3. Denton, J. J., Lederle Labs., U.S.A., Private Communication.
4. Uhlich, E., Univ. Munich, Germany, Private Communication.
5. Mitchell, G. M., Cardiff, U.K., Private Communication.
6. Hitzenberger, G., Univ. Vienna, Austria, (2 studies), Private
Communications.
7. Vrhovac, B., Univ. Zagreb, Yugoslavia, Private Communication.
8. Wayjen, R. G. A. van and Ende, A.v.d., Woerden, The
Netherlands, Private Communication.

RECEIVED August 21, 1978.

Etozolin: A Novel Diuretic

G. SATZINGER, M. HERRMANN, K.-O. VOLLMER, A. MERZWEILER,
and H. GOMAHR
Goedecke Research Institute, Goedecke AG, D-78 Freiburg (in Breisgau),
West Germany

O. HEIDENREICH and J. GREVEN
Pharmacological Department, Rhein.-Westf. Technical University of Aachen,
West Germany

Introduction - Investigations to date seem to indicate that
choleresis is, to some extent, part of the extrarenal effect of
diuretic substances. However, more detailed studies, particularly with furosemide and ethacrynic acid, have proved that
biliary osmolality is not affected hereby (1-4). The question
as to whether choleretics, which do not influence the biliary
electrolyte concentration, would make suitable models in the
search for novel diuretic substances has never been investigated. We have recently described (5) some highly potent
diuretic and well-tolerated compounds which were discovered in
the course of investigating a new class of heterocycles (Structure 1), many of which possess choleretic properties.

1

One of these compounds, ethyl Z-/3-methyl-4-oxo-5-(1-piper-
idinyl)-2-thiazolidinylidene/acetate (Compound 3, etozolin), has
been introduced as a therapeutic agent on the German market
under the trademark Elkapin. Table I summarizes the current
synthetic work in the field of 2-acylmethylene-4-thiazoli-
dinones. Table II shows the substitution pattern of the compounds of type 1 which are active diuretics. As a consequence
of these findings, six other series of heterocycles were synthesized and tested (Table III). None of the representatives of
these heterocycles exhibited diuretic activity, even when the
successful substitution pattern shown in Table II was employed
(as far as this was feasible and led to stable compounds).

0-8412-0464-0/78/47-083-**155**$09.00/0
© American Chemical Society

TABLE I

Synthesized and Tested Derivatives of 1

Substituent	Groups	Notes
R^1	H, alkyl, aralkyl, CH_2X, $(CH_2)_2X$	X = functional groups such as $-OR$, $-NR_2$, acyl (R = lower alkyl)
R^2	H, alkyl, aryl, aralkyl, CH_2X, $(CH_2)_2X$; $NHCOCH_3$; CO_2R	only for $R^3 = CH_3$
R^3	CH_3 $-CO_2H$, $-CO_2R$, $R-CO-$, $ArCO-$, $R-SO_2-$, $ArSO_2-$, $>NCO-$, $-HNCO-$, R_2NCO-, $-CN$; pyridyl, benzimidazolyl, indolyl	only for $R^2 = CO_2R$ AR = aryl, heteroaryl
R^4	H, alkyl, aryl $R^4/R^5 = >CR^2$	
R^5	$-N<$, $-N-N<$	aliph., arom., aliph.-arom., hetero-aliph. and arom. amines and hydrazines

TABLE II

Derivatives of 1 and Their Diuretic Activity
Relative to Etozolin (3)

Compound No.	R^1	R^2	R^3	R^4	R^5	Diuretic Activity (Relative to 3)
2	H	H	$CO_2C_2H_5$	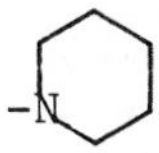 $-N\bigcirc$ (piperidino)	H	0.3
3	CH_3	H	$CO_2C_2H_5$	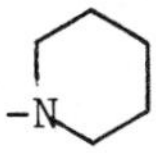 $-N\bigcirc$ (piperidino)	H	1.0
4	CH_3	H	CO_2CH_3	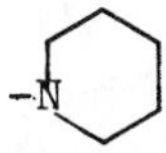 $-N\bigcirc$ (piperidino)	H	1.1
5	CH_3	H	CO_2H	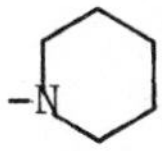 $-N\bigcirc$ (piperidino)	H	1.3
6	CH_3	H	CO_2H	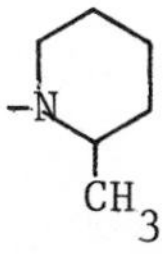 $-N\bigcirc$ (piperidino, CH_3)	H	0.6
7	CH_3	H	$CO_2C_2H_5$	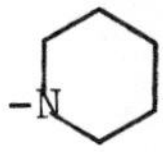 $-N\bigcirc$ (piperidino)	CH_3	0.1
8	CH_3	CH_3	$CO_2C_2H_5$	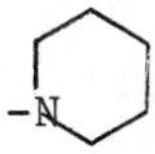 $-N\bigcirc$ (piperidino)	H	0.7
9	CH_3	$CO_2-C_2H_5$	CH_3	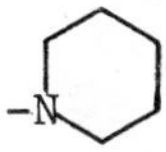 $-N\bigcirc$ (piperidino)	H	0.6
10	CH_3	H	$CO_2C_2H_5$	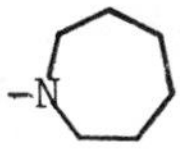 $-N\bigcirc$ (azepane)	H	0.6
11	CH_3	H	$\varnothing SO_2$	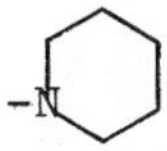 $-N\bigcirc$ (pyrrolidino)	H	0.5
12	CH_3	H	CH_3SO_2	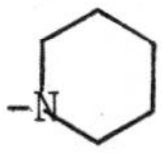 $-N\bigcirc$ (piperidino)	H	0.3

TABLE III

Schematic Representation of Heterocycles
Structurally Related to 1

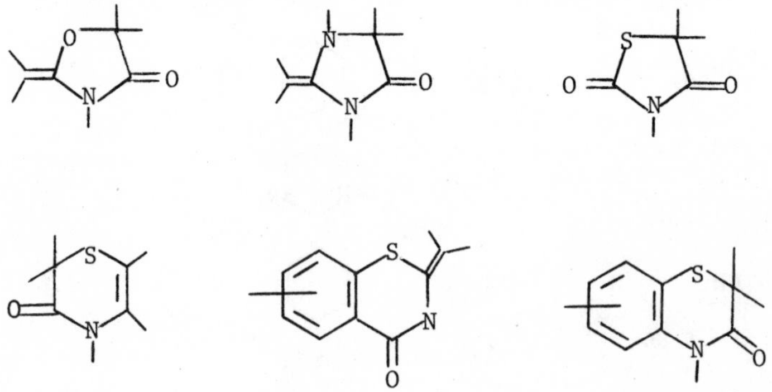

SAR of 2-Acylmethylene-4-Thiazolidinones - Changes in the substituent on the ring nitrogen (R^1) of compound 1 markedly affect diuretic activity. Even the change of R^1 = CH_3 to C_2H_5 leads to an abrupt loss of activity. Almost the same can be said of R^2 because activity is maintained only when R^2 = H or CH_3. Stereochemistry does not play an important role here since both the Z- and the E-isomer are active. Maximal activity is seen when R^3 is COOH or COOEt; the only other substituents allowed are methyl and phenylsulfonyl, and they produce less active compounds. Optimal activity is clearly achieved when R^4 is 1-piperidyl. Any enlargement or reduction of the ring size or any bridging or substitution reduces the activity and 2,6-disubstitution eliminates the activity. Introduction of a second substituent at C-5 (i.e., where R^5 is not H) does not lead to active compounds.

A particularly fascinating aspect is the homology of the most potent diuretic and choleretic substances, 3 and 13.

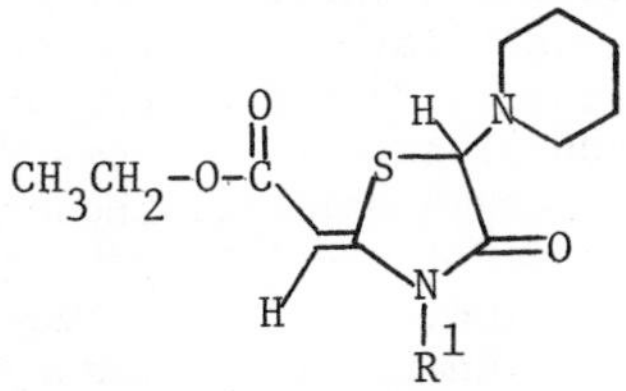

	R^1	
3	CH_3	etozolin
13	C_2H_5	piprozolin

However, as is illustrated below, compound 3 possesses only a very weak choleretic (side) effect and compound 13 has no diuretic effect. We investigated this phenomenon using spectroscopic, physical chemical and X-ray measurements. The spectroscopic and thermodynamic findings have been published (5), and some of the results of the X-ray studies will be discussed subsequently.

Comparison of 2-Acylmethylene-4-Thiazolidinones with Other Classes of Diuretics - As it will be discussed in detail below, the 2-acylmethylene-4-thiazolidinones represent a new class of high-ceiling diuretics to be added to the well known sulfamyl benzoic acids and acylphenoxyacetic acids. They all seem to have a similar effect on renal electrolyte transport. An examination of etozolin, furosemide and ethacrynic acid, each a representative of one of the three diuretic classes, reveals that they all have (a) the same main site of action (early distal tubular site) and (b) presumably, the same mechanism of action (inhibition of active chloride transport) (6-9).

At the present time, little is known about the mechanism of action of these diuretics; there are some indications that it involves inhibition of a renal adenyl cyclase (10). In order to develop working hypotheses on which to base an economical search

for new diuretics, it was of interest to investigate whether
these chemically different substances had some common structural
and/or electronic features. Such an approach seemed reasonable
considering the molecular rigidity of these classes of compounds. Figure 1 shows on the left the three classes of
high-ceiling diuretics: acylmethylene-4-thiazolidinones (14),
sulfamoylbenzoic acids (15) and acylphenoxyacetic acids (16).
The structural features thought to be important for activity are
delineated in the figure (11). On the right, the electronic
effects of these functional groups are indicated by the arrows;
the length and direction of the arrows reflect their relative
electron donor and acceptor properties. A striking feature is
the general pattern that appears whose dominant characteristics
are two groups with opposing electronic effects attached meta-
or para- to each other and linked by a ring system suitable for
the transmission of their electronic effects. The distances
between comparable charge centers (compound 3, 5-N/O-$\underline{C}$=O;
furosemide, N_{ar}/S; ethacrynic acid, 1-O/=C-$\underline{C}$-$\underline{C}$=O) are in the range
of 5.5-6.0 A. These distances were determined for compound 3,
from X-ray data, see below; furosemide, calculated from the data
of Price (12) and Dupont (13), ethacrynic acid data from Dreiding
models. X-ray analysis of compound 3 (detailed data on comparative X-ray analysis of the acylmethylene-4-thiazolidinones
will be published in a subsequent paper) furnishes interesting
information (Figure 2). The heterocycle, including the structural fragment shown below, is virtually planar. The symmetry
axis N/C-11 of the piperidine ring is approximately equatorial

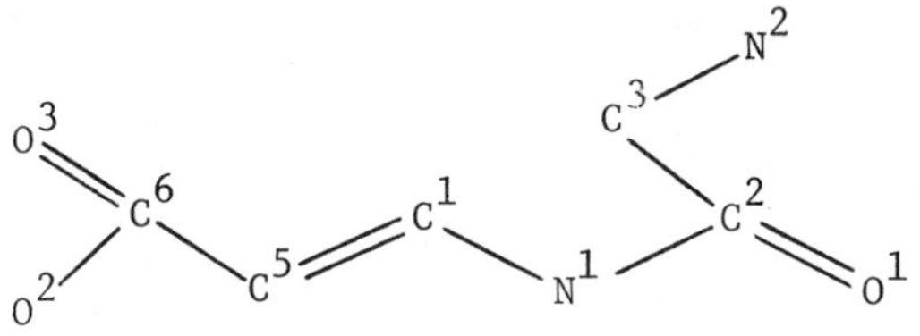

to this plane, and the averaged plane of the piperidine chair is
roughly vertical to it. The interatomic distances (Table IV) sub-
stantiate the inclusion of the ring sulfur S^1 in the electron
distribution of the whole planar system. In accordance with its
electronic situation and in contrast to the enone double bond of
the ethacrynic acid (19), the exocyclic double bond is not
nucleophilic; compound 3 does not react with sulfhydryl groups.
This fact does not contradict our argumentation because the
diuretic potency of the acylphenoxyacetic acids do not run parallel to the nucleophilic character of this bond (20).
    Analysis of the X-ray data furnishing some explanations for
the unusual SARs of the acylmethylene-4-thiazolidinones is as

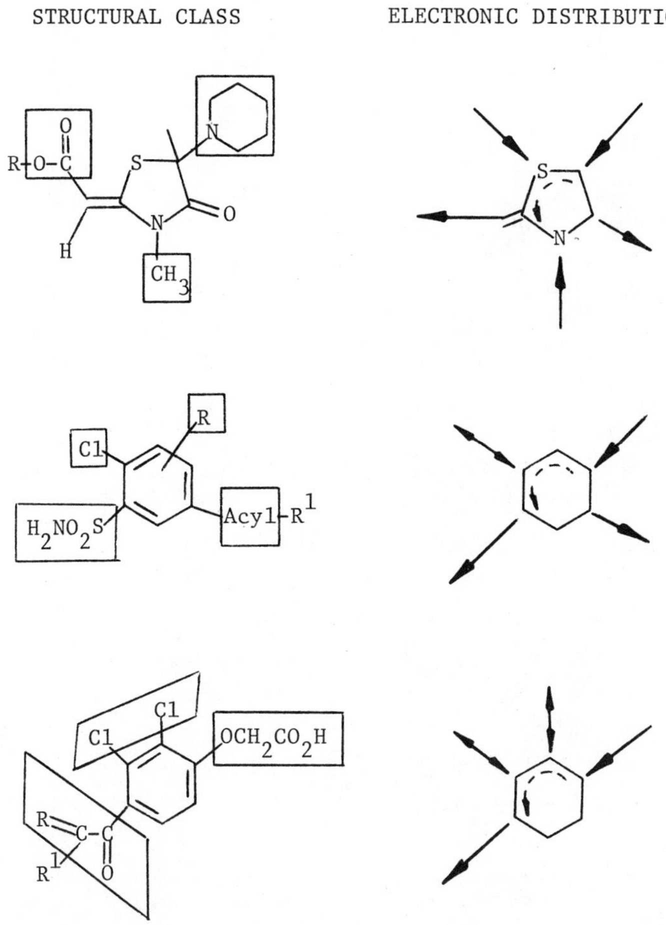

STRUCTURAL CLASS   ELECTRONIC DISTRIBUTION

14

15

16

Figure 1.   The three classes of high-ceiling diuretics with the moieties responsible for biological activity and their effects on electron distribution

Numbering

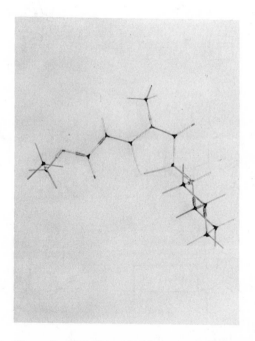

Figure 2. Dreiding Model of Compound 3 constructed on the basis of x-ray data. Viewed along the Z-axis (N_1: (0,0,0)). (The Dreiding model simulates plananty for the entire hetero ring not considering the deviation of S' by about 5°; thus, erroneously, 3-H is nearly eclipsed by C3-N2.)

TABLE IV

Characteristic Interatomic Distances and Bond
Angles of Compound 3 and their Anticipated Values

Etozolin (3) (Å)		Comparable Standard Values (Å)	Ref.
N2-C3	1.43	1.47 (aliphatic)	14
C3-S1	1.89	1.82 (aliphatic)	14
S1-C1	1.74	1.82 (aliphatic)	14
		1.72 (thiophene)	15
C1-C5	1.36	1.30 (acrylic acid)	16
C5-C6	1.41	1.47 (acrylic acid)	16
C6-O3	1.24	1.26 (acrylic acid)	16
C6-O2	1.34	1.28 (acrylic acid)	16
<C1-S1-C3	92°	91.9° (thiophene	15
		100-105° (aliphatic)	17
		105.5° (thiazolidine)	18

follows: 1) the exchange of the ring sulfur S^1 for other
heteroatoms or a change in its oxidation state should affect
or reduce its pseudo-aromatic state, 2) any increase in the size
of the substituent on the ring nitrogen beyond CH_3 should alter
the electron distribution in the molecule due to disturbance of
planarity or of hyperconjugation; the same applies to the steric
bulk and the nature of the acylmethylene group and 3) interaction between the piperidino nitrogen N^2 and the heterocyclic
ring is dependent on the former's unhindered spatial flexi-
bility. Other influences are probably attributable to the
effects of the 5-amino group on transport (5).

PHARMACOLOGY

Acute Toxicity - The acute toxicity of etozolin was studied
in male mice (NMRI) and rats (SIV 50). The calculation of the
LD_{50} values was based on the probit analysis according to Weber
(21). The results are shown in Table V.

TABLE V

Acute Toxicity of Etozolin in Mice and Rats
Following i.g. and i.p. Administration

Species	Sex	Route of Adminis- tration	LD_{50} (mg/kg)	Confidence Limits p = 0.05 (mg/kg)	
				lower	upper
Mouse	male	i.g.	8,670	7,310	10,270
Mouse	female	i.g.	9,360	7,290	12,030
Mouse	male	i.p.	1,210	1,093	1,340
Rat	male	i.g.	11,040	9,380	13,000
Rat	female	i.g.	10,250	9,260	11,350
Rat	male	i.p.	1,575	1,355	1,830

As the values shown in Table V indicate, the acute i.g. and i.p.
toxicity of etozolin is extremely low. The LD_{50} values did not
show any appreciable difference in male or female animals. The
toxicity of the compound is slightly less in rats than in mice.
The low p.o. toxicity of the drug was also confirmed in a pilot
dose range-finding study in dogs. In this species, the first
evidence of toxicity occurred at 1,600 mg/kg; at 3,200 mg/kg,
the lower lethal dose range was reached.
Diuretic Activity - Clearance Tests in Dogs: These studies
served to reveal the diuretic effect of etozolin as the hydrochloride salt in female dogs weighing between 10 and 29 kg (22).

The doses administered i.v. ranged from 6 to 100 mg/kg. The animals were anesthetized by means of an i.v. injection of 30 mg/kg pentobarbital sodium (Nembutal$_R$). In order to fill the extracellular space with a sufficient fluid, 25 ml/kg isotonic saline solution was infused i.v. within one hour followed by continuous i.v. administration of fluid at a rate of 2 ml/min to which enough creatinine and PAH were added to achieve and maintain constant plasma levels of about 20 mg % and 1.5 mg %, respectively. After a one-hour period of equilibration, the urine was collected during 10 to 20 min periods by means of a catheter. In the middle of each period, blood was withdrawn from the femoral artery. Na^+, K^+ and Cl^- as well as creatinine and PAH were measured in blood and urine. Furthermore, the urinary output and the urine pH were recorded. The first diuretic effects were noted at about 20 mg/kg and reached almost maximal values at 50 mg/kg. Table VI shows a typical result after i.v. administration of 50 mg/kg. The diuretic effect of etozolin reached its peak within 1 hour after i.v. injection. As in the other studies, there was a slight decrease in creatinine clearance, which is used as a measure of GFR in dogs. PAH clearance rates dropped to one-third or even less in each trial and, thus, approached the creatinine clearance values. This signified that the drug interfered with PAH secretion in the proximal tubule, so that PAH clearance could not be used to measure renal plasma flow following administration of this agent. The maximum tubular transport capacity for PAH (Tm_{PAH}) was determined in four separate studies. After i.v. injection of 50 mg/kg of etozolin, the mean Tm_{PAH} value fell from 7.28 to 1.76 mg/min. Both the urinary electrolyte excretion and total urinary output increased by multiples of their original values following administration of 50 mg/kg of etozolin and chloride excretion consistently exceeded that of sodium. The most reliable indicator of the potency of a diuretic, independent of body weight, is its percentage of inhibition of electrolyte reabsorption. In the example illustrated in Table VI, sodium reabsorption fell to 83% and chloride reabsorption dropped to 80%. Tubular potassium reabsorption also decreased, although no excretion levels were measured which were more than twice the baseline values. Urine pH was lower in all the tests than in the control periods, indicating an increase in hydrogen ion secretion.

The next studies were concerned with experimental changes in pH. Alkalosis was induced by i.v. infusion of an $NaHCO_3$ solution and acidosis by infusion of 0.1 N HCl. The action of etozolin was severely inhibited by metabolic alkalosis but was essentially unaffected by acidosis.

In a series of 18 tests involving 8 female dogs weighing 15 to 30 kg, a study was conducted to determine whether etozolin potentiates the effect of chlorothiazide and/or chlormerodrin, or conversely, whether peak chlorothiazide or chlormerodrin .

TABLE VI

Effect of Etozolin (50 mg/kg) i.v. on Renal Function of a Female Dog of 17 kg

Time	Urine flow	GFR (C_creat)	C_{PAH}	Urinary Excretion			Fractional Reabsorption			pH
				Na^+	K^+	Cl^-	Na^+	K^+	Cl^-	
min		ml/min		micro Eq/min			%			Urine
-20-10	3.0	68	269	435	72	420	95.6	67.1	95.6	7.30
-10- 0	2.1	59	221	292	65	285	96.5	67.0	96.5	7.27
0				50 mg/kg Etozolin						
10-30	5.4	48	75	810	108	853	88.1	32.1	87.3	6.71
30-50	8.0	45	69	1088	136	1233	83.0	3.5	80.4	6.70
50-70	7.6	52	64	981	129	1102	86.9	20.4	85.0	6.82
70-90	6.5	40	57	793	117	929	86.5	7.1	83.0	6.87
90-110	5.8	46	55	684	105	794	89.6	26.6	87.7	6.73
110-130	4.7	42	52	554	94	653	89.3	36.5	89.2	6.67
130-150	4.7	36	54	550	89	625	89.5	23.9	87.4	6.59

diuresis can be enhanced by this agent (23). Etozolin was found to have an additive effect on the maximum Na^+, Cl^- and K^+ excretion and urinary output produced by chlorothiazide and by chlormerodrin. Likewise, chlorothiazide and chlormerodrin enhanced the diuresis produced by etozolin. With the test methods used, it was not possible to establish whether these results were due to the three diuretics having different mechanisms of action or different sites of action in the nephron.

Micropuncture Studies in Rats - The object of performing diuretic studies in rats was to investigate the effect of etozolin in another species (22,24). First, dose-response curves were generated and then attempts were made to locate the site of action in the nephron using micropuncture techniques (25). Figure 3 shows the effect of i.g. administration of the drug in comparison to furosemide on the four-hour urinary output and Na^+, Cl^- and K^+ elimination, calculated as output per kg of body weight. Etozolin and furosemide were intubated orally as 1% tragacanth suspensions which were diluted with 0.2% saline solution. The controls received the same volume of tragacanth but without the diuretic. All the animals were then administered 40 ml/kg of a 0.2% saline solution i.g., so that the total volume of fluid intubated equaled 5% of the body weight. The test groups consisted of 8 to 12 animals which were kept in separate diuresis cages.

Both etozolin and furosemide had dose-related diuretic effects, furosemide being obviously the more potent of the two. Each compound produced a greater increase in chloride excretion than in sodium excretion. This tendency seemed to be somewhat more pronounced for etozolin than for furosemide.

Micropuncture Data - On the basis of the dose-response curves, an i.v. dose of 50 mg/kg of etozolin was selected for the micropuncture studies. Male anesthetized Sprague-Dawley rats were used. The animals were prepared for micropuncture in the usual way (25). Two to three late proximal and early distal punctures were made, and the drug was injected i.v. After an interval of 30 min, two to three more late proximal and early distal tubular segments were micropunctured. The tubular fluid was collected quantitatively and the inulin, sodium and potassium concentrations were determined. Table VII shows the micropuncture data for the late proximal nephron segments. Transit time was found to be extended after the administration of etozolin. None of the other parameters measured in the proximal convoluted tubule was significantly affected. Table VIII contains the micropuncture data of the early distal nephron segments.

Etozolin caused a pronounced increase in the flow rate of tubular fluid in the early distal tubular segments, a decrease in the TF/P-inulin ratio, an increase in sodium and potassium concentration and a rise in the TF/P-sodium and TF/P-potassium ratios. Fluid and electrolyte reabsorption in the loop of Henle

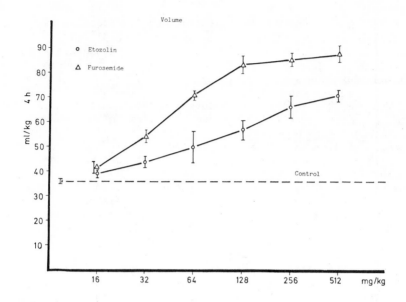

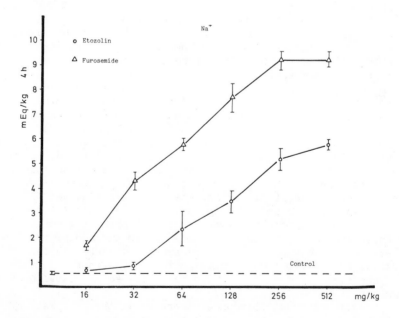

*Figure 3. Comparison of the dose–response curves of etozolin and furose-
mide after i.g. administration to rats. Urinary output and Na⁺ (top), Cl⁻ and
K⁺ (right) excretion over a four-hour period are shown (x ± sₓ, n = 8). The
dotted lines represent the control values (x ± sₓ, n = 32).*

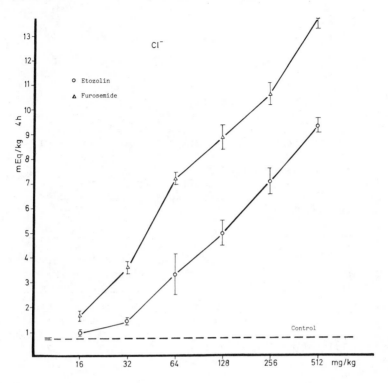

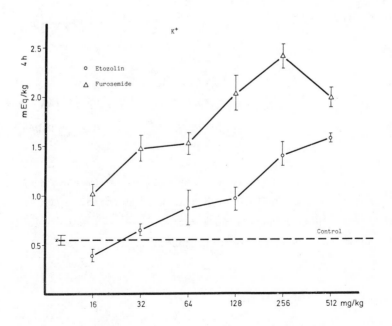

170

DIURETIC AGENTS

TABLE VII

Summary of the micropuncture data obtained by measurement at the end of the proximal convoluted tubules of
superficial nephrons. Transit time is the time from
the diffuse coloration of the kidney surface after
lissamine green injection until the dye columns
converge into the terminal portions of the proximal
convolution.

	Control	Etozolin 50 mg/kg i.v. stat; then, 50 mg/kg/h i.v.
Transit Time (sec)	7.53 + 0.37 n = 6/12	10.8 + 0.86* n = 6/11
Nephron Filtration Rate (nl/min)	27.9 + 3.6 n = 7/11	22.3 + 2.7 n = 6/10
Flow Rate (nl/min)	10.3 + 0.7 n = 8/12	9.6 + 0.9 n = 7/12
$\frac{TF}{P}$ inulin	2.68 + 0.27 n = 7/12	2.49 + 0.37 n = 6/10
$\frac{TF}{P}$ Na^+	1.02 + 0.02 n = 7/12	0.99 + 0.02 n = 8/11
$\frac{TF}{P}$ K^+	1.04 + 0.05 n = 7/12	0.97 + 0.04 n = 8/11

Mean $\pm$ S.E.M.; n = number of animals/number of measurements;
$\frac{TF}{P}$ Inulin = tubular fluid to plasma inulin ratio; $\frac{TF}{P}$ Na^+ =
tubular fluid to plasma sodium ratio; $\frac{TF}{P}$ K^+ = tubular fluid
to plasma potassium ratio; nl = nanoliters; *p <0.01.

TABLE VIII

Summary of the Micropuncture Data Obtained by
Measurement at the Early Distal Tubular Site

	Control	Etozolin 50 mg/kg i.v., stat; then, 50 mg/kg/h i.v.
Nephron Filtration Rate (nl/min)	28.0 ± 2.9 n = 6/11	25.2 ± 4.4 n = 5/9
Flow Rate (nl/min)	6.0 ± 0.9 n = 6/11	8.9 ± 1.0* n = 5/9
$\frac{TF}{P}$ Inulin	4.98 ± 0.73 n = 6/11	2.72 ± 0.30* n = 5/9
Early Distal Sodium Concentration (mEq/L)	42.4 ± 3.5 n = 6/11	78.5 ± 8.5** n = 5/9
Early Distal Potassium Concentration (mEq/L)	1.12 ± 0.09 n = 6/11	2.52 ± 0.41** n = 5/9
$\frac{TF}{P}$ Na^+	0.274 ± 0.037 n = 6/11	0.543 ± 0.048** n = 5/9
$\frac{TF}{P}$ K^+	0.270 ± 0.031 n = 6/11	0.615 ± 0.074** n = 5/9

Mean ± S.E.M.; n = number of animals/number of measurements; $\frac{TF}{P}$ Inulin = tubular fluid to plasma inulin ratio; $\frac{TF}{P}$ Na^+ = tubular fluid to plasma sodium ratio; $\frac{TF}{P}$ K^+ = tubular fluid to plasma potassium ratio; *p <0.01; nl = nanoliters; **p <0.001.

can be calculated from the late proximal and early distal data.
Under the influence of the drug, fluid reabsorption in this
nephron segment fell from 41.7 to 7.3%, sodium reabsorption from
82.9 to 48.7% and potassium reabsorption from 83.3 to 36%. It
can be concluded from these findings that diuretic and natriuretic action of etozolin derives from the substance's inhibition of fluid and electrolyte reabsorption in the loop of Henle.

The major metabolite of etozolin, (Z)-β-methyl-4-oxo-5-(1-
piperidinyl)-2-thiazolidinylidene⁷acetic acid, was also subjected
to detailed pharmacological investigation. It possesses potent
diuretic properties and its site of action is also located in
the ascending limb of Henle's loop. All the results suggest
that this metabolite plays a major part in the biological
activity observed for etozolin.

General Pharmacology - Extensive pharmacological screening
did not reveal any results which were not attributable to the
diuretic action of etozolin. The chemical relationship of this
substance to known active choleretic compounds prompted us to
undertake studies to compare etozolin and piprozolin (Compound
13) in rats. Piprozolin was also evaluated for diuretic activity in rats. Conscious animals weighing 160 to 200 g were
employed. They were administered the test substance together
with 5 ml/100 g body weight of a 0.2% saline solution and the
urine was collected over a 4 hour period. Rats weighing 200 to
250 g, anesthetized with pentobarbital were used for the choleresis tests. The effluent bile was measured for 120 minutes
with a drop counter. The results of these studies are presented
in Figures 4 and 5.

Despite the close chemical relationship of the two compounds, etozolin showed only a slight choleretic action compared
to piprozolin. While 100 mg/kg of piprozolin caused a rapid
increase in bile secretion lasting over 90 minutes, only a
slight, slow increase in bile secretion was observed after
etozolin. Even 250 mg/kg of etozolin produced a marginal increase which subsided after 60 minutes, while 200 mg/kg of
piprozolin had a stronger dose-related effect than did 100
mg/kg. While 50, 100 and 200 mg/kg of etozolin administered
intragastrically caused a dose-related increase in urine elimination, piprozolin showed no significant effect at the same
doses.

An important factor in long-term treatment with diuretics is
their effect on glucose metabolism. Therefore, corresponding
glucose tolerance tests were conducted in connection with the
long-term experiments in rats and dogs (26). In rats, the
dosages were 50, 250 and 2,000 mg/kg/day; the duration of the
experiment was 18 months. Oral doses of 30, 120 and 480 mg/kg/-
day were administered to dogs for 12 months. A glucose tolerance test was conducted in dogs after the 1st, 4th, 8th, 12th,
26th, 39th and 52nd week and in rats after the 26th and 78th
week. Two g of glucose/kg of body weight were administered as a

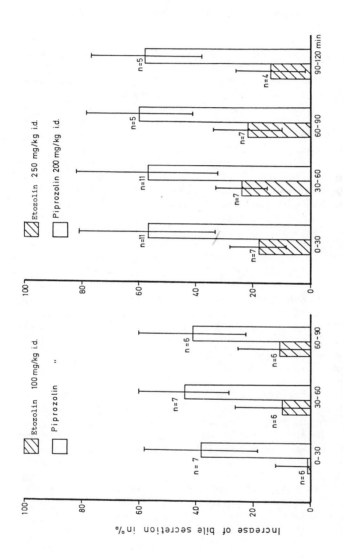

Figure 4. Effect of etozolin (100 and 250 mg/kg) and piprozolin (100 and 200 mg/kg) on bile secretion in anesthetized rats following i.d. administration

20% solution via a stomach tube. Following an 18 hour food
abstinence period, serum glucose was measured before administration and then 1 hour and 4 hours after administration of the
drug. There were no differences between the animals treated and
the controls at any time during the experiment. Thus, the
possibility of glucose intolerance in rats and dogs can be
excluded even when high doses of etozolin are given over long
periods of time.

   Antihypertensive Effects in Rats - The antihypertensive
properties of etozolin were tested in conscious rats with
hypertension of different origin: (a) induced by desoxy-
corticosterone acetate (DOCA), (b) hereditary and (c) reno-
vascular hypertension caused by experimental impairment of the
renal circulation. Blood pressure was measured non-invasively
at the base of the tail either via a condenser microphone or
plethysmographically. Etozolin was administered intragastrically suspended in 1% tragacanth via a stomach tube once a
day. The results of these tests are shown in Figures 6, 7 and
8. As we had expected, the most pronounced effects were observed in the DOCA-treated rats, since the impaired sodium
balance was restored to its normal level and the volume of
extracellular fluid was reduced as a result of the diuretic
action of etozolin. The blood pressure was also significantly
lowered in rats with renovascular hypertension and in animals
with spontaneous hypertension. Since the three types of hypertension are caused by different mechanisms, there is reason to
believe that the antihypertensive effect of etozolin derives not
only from a reduction of the plasma volume, but also from
peripheral mechanisms, possibly of the same kind as are postu-
lated for the thiazides.

METABOLISM AND PHARMACOKINETICS

   The fate of etozolin in the organism was investigated using
^{14}C-etozolin labeled in the 2-position of the thiazolidine ring
(27). The absorption of ^{14}C-etozolin was $\geq$ 90% in man, $\geq$ 80% in
rats and to a lesser degree in dogs. In all species, maximum
^{14}C blood levels were observed 2 to 3 hours after oral administration. After 24 hours, the concentration of radioactive
material in the blood had dropped to approximately 8% of the
maximum values in rats and dogs and to approximately 15% in man.
In rats, the blood levels can be described by a one-compartment
body model, the absorption half-life being approximately 0.6
hour, and the elimination half-life being approximately 6 hours.
During absorption, etozolin underwent a distinct first-pass
effect. In all species, the majority of the plasma radioactivity corresponded to metabolite I (see Figure 9), which also
has diuretic activity. Unchanged drug appeared in plasma in
considerably lower concentrations. In rats, more than 90% of
plasma radioactivity could be ascribed to metabolite I. In man,

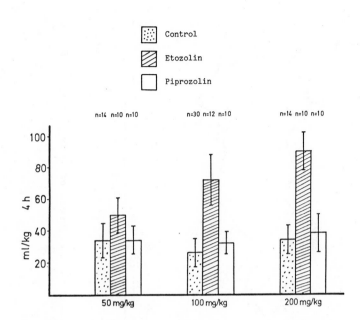

Figure 5.   Effect of increasing doses of etozolin and piprozolin on urine excretion in conscious rats

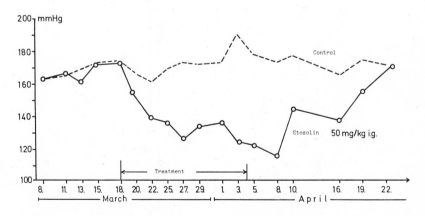

Figure 6.   Effect of 50 mg/kg etozolin i.g. on DOCA-induced hypertension in rats: 19 drug treated animals; 10 control animals

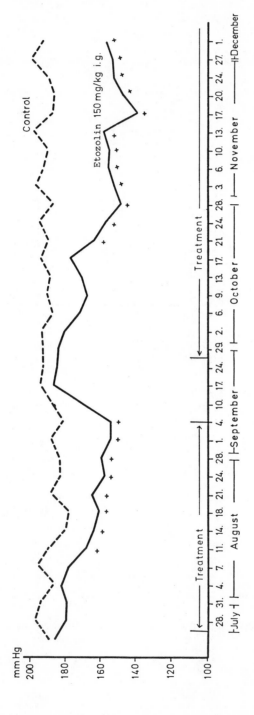

Figure 7. Effect of repeated i.g. treatment with 150 mg/kg of etozolin on the blood pressure of rats with spontaneous hypertension,
$+ = p \geq 0.05$

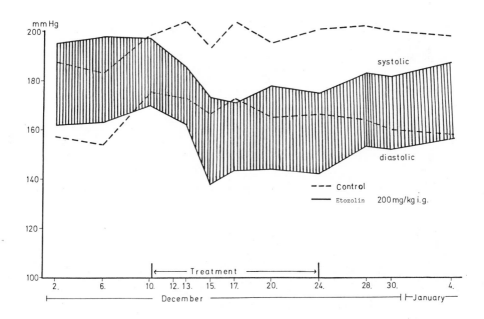

Figure 8. Effect of etozolin on systolic and diastolic blood pressure in rats with reno-vascular hypertension. Experimental and control groups consisted of 10 animals each.

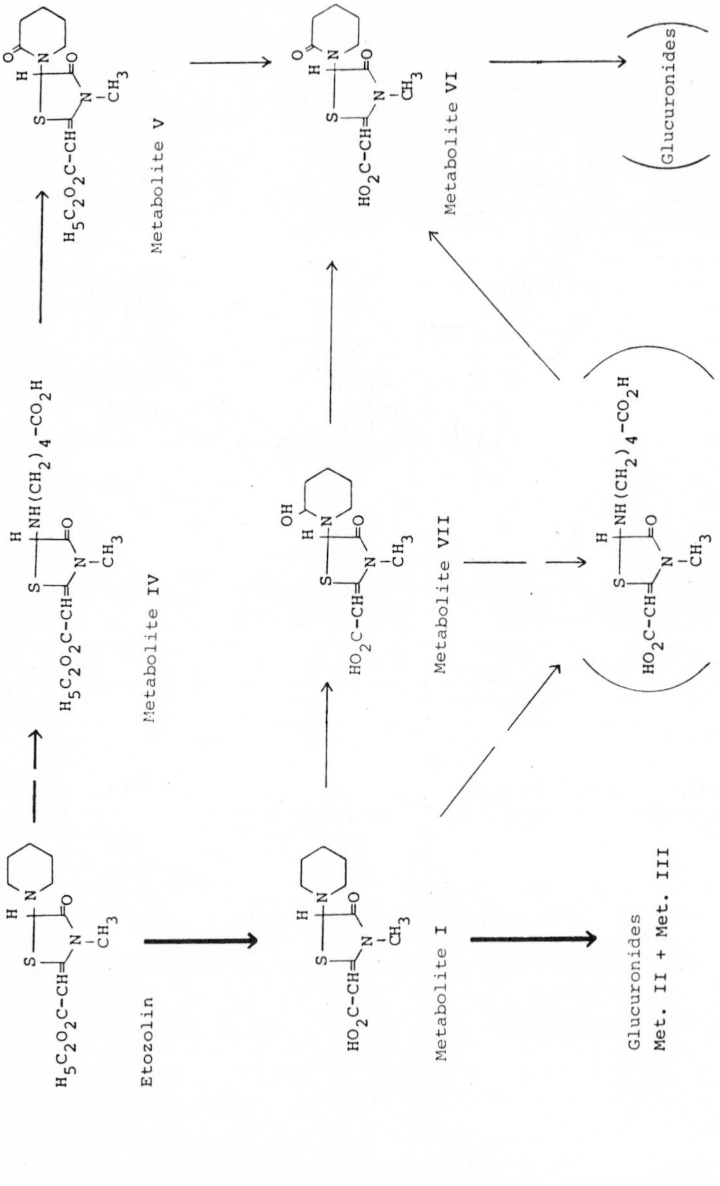

Figure 9. Proposed metabolic pathway of etozolin in rats, dogs, and man

approximately 80% corresponded to the sum of metabolite I and the unchanged drug during the 0 to 8 hour observation period. In all species, the main portion of the blood radioactivity was present in the plasma. In vitro investigation of human plasma revealed a low protein binding for etozolin and metabolite I (approximately 45% and 35%, respectively).

In rats, approximately 80% of the radioactivity was eliminated in the urine and the half-life was 6 hours; in man approximately 90% was eliminated in the urine and the half-life was 8.5 hours. The renal ^{14}C elimination in dogs ranged between 29% and 72%. In man, almost 100% of the radioactive dose was recovered in the excrement within four days. In rats, the highest ^{14}C concentrations were found in blood, kidneys and liver. In the other organs, the concentrations were generally much lower, the lowest being in the brain (27). Autoradiography of rats following repeated oral administration of 100 mg of ^{14}C-etozolin/kg/day from the 10-17 day of pregnancy revealed substantially lower radioactivity concentrations in the fetuses than in the mothers (28). The radioactivity was distributed uniformly throughout the fetal organs, the lowest concentrations occurring in the brain. The placenta would appear to act as a barrier, restricting the passage of radioactive compounds from the mother's circulation into the fetal tissue. The structures of the metabolites were elucidated in studies using rat, dog and human urine and rat bile obtained after oral administration of ^{14}C-etozolin (29). Seven metabolites were isolated. The metabolic pathway of etozolin is the same in rats, dogs and man, and is characterized in three steps (Figure 9): 1) enzymatic cleavage of the ester group, which leads to the main metabolite (metabolite I) in the plasma of all 3 species, 2) glucuronidation of the resulting metabolite I, leading to metabolites II and III, which are diastereoisomeric esters of the two enantiomeric forms of metabolite I with β-D-glucuronic acid and 3) oxidation of the piperidine moiety to metabolites IV-VII.

In all species, approximately 50-60% of the urinary radioactivity corresponded to the sum of the free metabolite I and the metabolite I glucuronides. The unconjugated form was more abundant in rats, while the metabolite I glucuronides predominated in man. Intermediate results were obtained using dogs. No unchanged substance was found in the urine of any of the species investigated. There was little variance in the excretion ratios and urinary metabolite profiles in rats following the oral intubation of different doses (3-100 mg/kg) of the drug, indicating that etozolin's metabolism is not dose related in this range.

A specific TLC analytical method was used to study the pharmacokinetics of the unchanged substance and its principal metabolite (metabolite I) following single and repeated administration of various doses by different routes (30). The pharmacokinetic behavior of etozolin and metabolite I could be

described by first-order process models in each study. Etozolin
was metabolized fairly rapidly in each of the species investigated, only relatively low concentrations being found in plasma
and none in urine. No deep compartment distribution (e.g.,
protein binding) was detected. Minor differences were observed
in the excretion of the principal metabolite (half-life 4-8
hours), but the uniform distribution volume of approximately 1
L/kg indicates that the metabolite's apparent volume of distribution is identical in all three species.

Each species was administered a different dose range. The
pharmacokinetic behavior of etozolin and its principal metabolite was not dose related in the ranges investigated (5-50 mg/kg
i.v. in rats, 30-480 mg/kg i.g. in dogs, 400-800 mg orally in
man). The plasma level time-curves for etozolin and metabolite
I in man are shown in Figure 10.

Etozolin was investigated in long-term studies in man and
dogs. The human study involved patients with impaired renal
function. The pharmacokinetics of etozolin and metabolite I
were unaffected by the size of the multiple doses given. It has
been demonstrated that neither the parent substance nor metabolite I is likely to accumulate in the organism if the recommended therapeutic dosage intervals are observed.

CLINICAL STUDIES

   Comparative Studies of the Diuretic Activity in Normal
Volunteers - The diuretic effect of etozolin was first investigated in 8 healthy volunteers (31). A clear dose-dependent
diuretic effect could be demonstrated. When compared to mefruside as a reference substance, both compounds showed a similar
diuretic profile. The maximum effect occurred 2 to 4 hours
after oral administration; the duration of the increased diuresis being about 10 hours. However, at the doses used, the
total volume excreted was significantly higher with etozolin
than with mefruside (Figure 11).

The diuretic profile of etozolin is different from that of
furosemide, as shown by the total urinary output after equi-
effective doses. Furosemide, in contrast to etozolin and the
thiazide diuretics, has a very rapid onset of diuresis, lasting
about 2 hours with a rapid decrease in urine output followed by
a distinct rebound phenomenon lasting over 12 hours (Figures 12,
13, 14).

   Antihypertensive Activity - In a controlled trial in patients with essential hypertension, 200 mg of etozolin or half
the diuretic dose showed an antihypertensive effect similar to
that of a drug combination consisting of 150.0 mg of inositol
nicotinate + 15 mg mefruside + 0.15 mg reserpine (Figure 15).

In another controlled study (32), lasting over 6 months, a
pronounced antihypertensive effect could be observed (Figure
16).

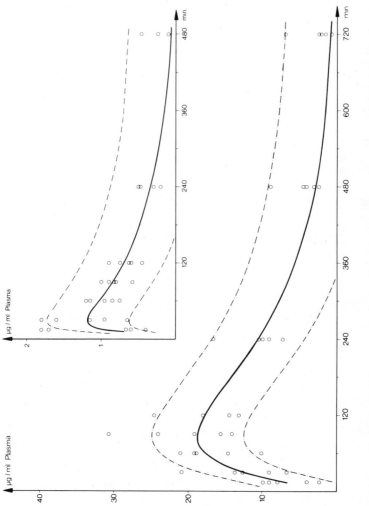

Figure 10. Plasma level time curves of the unchanged drug (top right) and metabolite I (bottom) after oral administration of 800 mg of etozolin to man. The 95% confidence interval of the function and the measured plasma level concentrations are also shown.

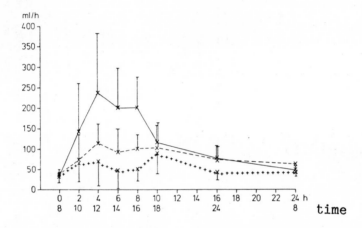

Figure 11. Mean value of urine volume. (——) Etozolin, 800 mg,
n = 8; (– – –) mefruside, 50 mg, n = 8; (+ +) placebo, n = 8.

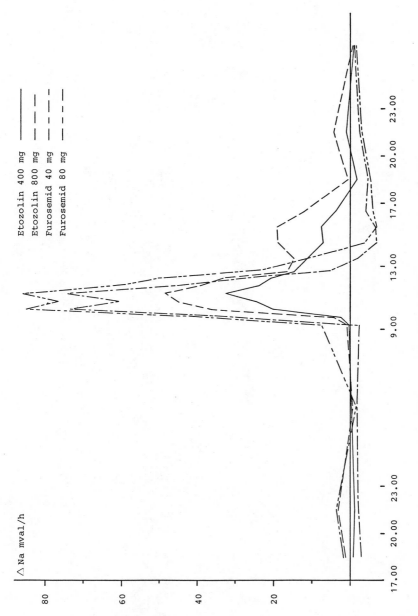

Figure 12.   Dose and drug-dependent urinary excretion of sodium

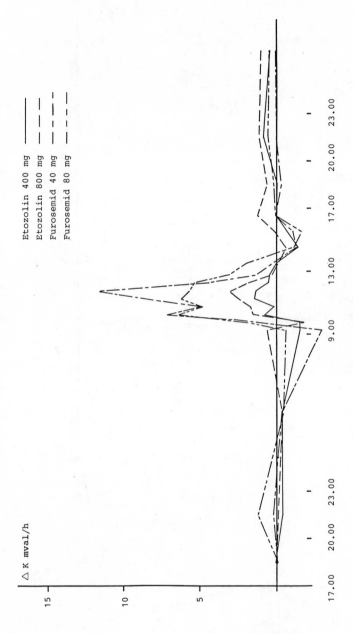

Figure 13.   Dose and drug-dependent urinary excretion of potassium

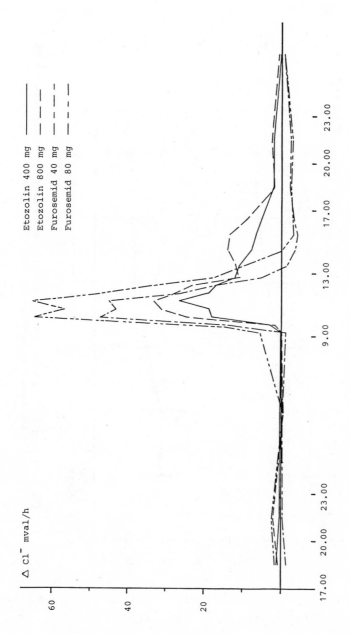

Figure 14. Dose and drug-dependent urinary excretion of chloride

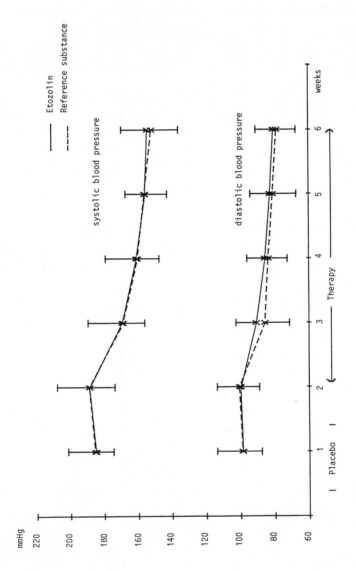

Figure 15.   Curves of mean blood pressure values in a sitting position during six months therapy with etozolin and with a reference substance (combination)

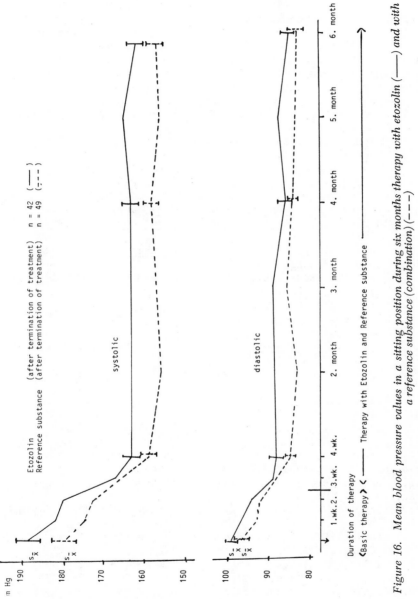

Figure 16. Mean blood pressure values in a sitting position during six months therapy with etozolin (———) and with a reference substance (combination) (– – –)

Side Effects - Out of 447 patients with edema of varying
etiology, 29 (6.49%) reported side effects: nausea, 2.0%;
vomiting, 1.6%; dizziness, 0.2%; headache, 0.7%; gastrointes-
tinal complaints, 0.9%; skin rashes, 0.9%. Some patients
complained of two or more side effects. It is yet to be
established whether these side effects are attributable to
etozolin alone since other drugs were administered concomi-
tantly. The characteristic side effects of diuretic and/or
hypotensive therapy, i.e., hyperuricemia and elevation of
creatinine levels also occurred with etozolin.

Literature Cited

1. Clodi, P. H. and Schnack, H., _Wiener klin. Wschr._, (1966),
78, 774.
2. Campese, V. M. and Siro-Brigiani, G., _Boll. Soc. Ital.
biol. sperim._, (1971), **47**, 22.
3. Maxwell, D. R., Szwed, J. J., Hamburger, R. J., Yu., P.
and Kleit, S. A., _Am. J. Physiol._, (1974), **226**, 540.
4. Heintze, K., Gotz, R. and Koerlings, H., _Naunyn-
Schmiedeberg's Arch. Pharm._, (1977), **297** (Suppl. 2), 150.
5. Satzinger, G., _Arzneim.-Forsch./Drug Research_, (1977), **27**,
(9a), 1742.
6. Greven, J. and Heidenreich, O., _Arzneim.-Forsch./Drug
Research_, (1977), **27**, (9a), 1755.
7. Burg, M., Stoner, L., Cardinal, J. and Green, N., _Am. J.
Physiol._, (1973), **225**, 119.
8. Burg, M. and Green, N., _Kidney Int._, (1973), **4**, 301.
9. Jacobson, H. R. and Kokko, J. H., _Ann. Rev. Pharm._,
(1976), **16**, 201.
10. Ebel, H., _Naunyn-Schmiedeberg's Arch. Pharm._, (1974), **281**,
301.
11. Meng, K. and Loew, D., "Diuretika", pp. 3,7,8,11, Georg
Thieme, Stuttgart, 1974.
12. Price, C. C. and Oae, S., "Sulfur Bonding", p. 61, Ronald,
N. Y., 1962.
13. Dupont, L. and Dideberg, O., _Acta Cryst._, (1972), **B28**,
2340.
14. Yukawa, Y., "Handbook of Organic Structural Analysis", pp.
518, 519, W. A. Benjamin Inc., N. Y., 1965.
15. Harshbarger, W. R. and Bauer, S. H., _Acta Cryst._, (1970),
B26, 1010.
16. Higgs, M. A. and Sass, R. L., _Acta Cryst._, (1963), **16**,
657.
17. Pauling, L., "Die Natur der chemischen Bindung", p. 108,
Verlag Chemie, Weinheim/Bergstrasse, 1962.
18. Miller, R. A. L., Robertson, J. M., Sim, G. A., Clapp, R.
C., Long, L. and Hasselstrom, T., _Nature_, (1964), **202**, 287.
19. Gunther, T. and Ahlers, J., _Arzneim. Forsch./Drug
Research_, (1976), **26**, (1), 13.

20. Schultz, E. M., Smith, R. L. and Woltersdorf, O. W., Jr., Ann. Rep. Med. Chem., (1975), 10, 71.
21. Weber, E., "Grundri der biologischen Statistik", p. 582, Gustav Fischer Verlag, Jena, 1972.
22. Heidenreich, O., Gharemani, G., Keller, P., Kook, Y. and Schmiz, K., Arzneim.-Forsch./Drug Research, (1964), 14, 1242.
23. Heidenreich, O. and Baumeister, L., Klin. Wschr., (1964), 42, 1236.
24. Herrmann, M., Bahrmann, H., Birkenmayer, E., Ganser, V., Heldt, W. and Steinbrecher, W., Arzneim.-Forsch./Drug Research, (1977), 27, 1745.
25. Greven, J. and Heidenreich, O., Arzneim.-Forsch./Drug Research, (1977), 27, 1755.
26. Herrmann, M., Wiegleb, J. and Leuschner, F., Arzneim.-Forsch./Drug Research, (1977), 27, 1758.
27. Vollmer, K.-O., v. Hodenberg, A., Poisson, A., Gladigau, V. and Hengy, H., Arzneim.-Forsch./Drug Research, (1977), 27, 1767.
28. Franklin, E. R., Chasseaud, L. F. and Taylor, T., Arzneim. Forsch/Drug Research, (1977), 27, 1800.
29. V. Hodenberg, A., Vollmer, K.-O., Klemisch, W. and Liedtke, B., Arzneim.-Forsch./Drug Research, (1977), 27, 1776.
30. Gladigau, V. and Vollmer, K.-O., Arzneim.-Forsch./Drug Research, (1977), 27, 1786.
31. Biamino, G., Arzneim.-Forsch./Drug Research, (1977), 27, 1814.
32. Felix, G., Windsheimer, F. and Otrzonsek, G.. Private Communication.

RECEIVED August 21, 1978.

11

The Evolution of the (Aryloxy)acetic Acid Diuretics

O. W. WOLTERSDORF, JR., S. J. DE SOLMS, and E. J. CRAGOE, JR.

Merck Sharp and Dohme Research Laboratories, West Point, PA 19486

The advent of modern diuretic therapy occurred with the discovery of the diuretic properties of merbaphen (1, 2). In spite of the tremendous advances in the field, the mercurial diuretics, particularly the phenoxyacetic acids, merbaphen (Compound 1, Figure 1) and mersalyl (Compound 2, Figure 1) possess many pharmacodynamic attributes which are as good as, or superior to, the modern agents, including potent saluresis, proper urinary Na^+/Cl^- balance, an acceptable potassium excretion profile and uricosuric activity. In addition, much is known concerning their mechanism of action. Cafruny(3) and others have shown that the mercurials react with sulfhydryl-containing compounds both in vitro and in vivo and that such a reaction at the renal receptor is associated with the observed saluresis and diuresis. Also, the concentration of protein-bound sulfhydryl groups in renal cells is minimal when the concentration of mercury is maximal, which is also the time when diuresis is maximal.

The advantages of the mercurials were more than outweighed by their disadvantages which included tachyphylaxis, poor oral efficacy and toxicity. Using the mercurial phenoxyacetic acids as models, a search was initiated in our laboratories by J. M. Sprague and co-workers for a non-mercurial agent which would lack the drawbacks of the mercurials but would possess their diuretic properties.

Our approach to the solution of this problem was to search for a chemical moiety that would mimic the chemical behavior of the mercury atom in the diuretic mercurials, especially as it pertains to reactions with sulfhydryl groups. After a long investigation, the α,β-unsaturated ketones (3) were found to react by a Michael-type reaction with standard sulfhydryl-containing substances in a parallel fashion to mercurials (4) even under physiological conditions of pH and temperature as shown by the two equations in Figure 2.

Acryloylbenzoic acids of the type 3 were known at the time, but when synthesized proved to be inactive as diuretics. This

0-8412-0464-0/78/47-083-**190**$10.25/0

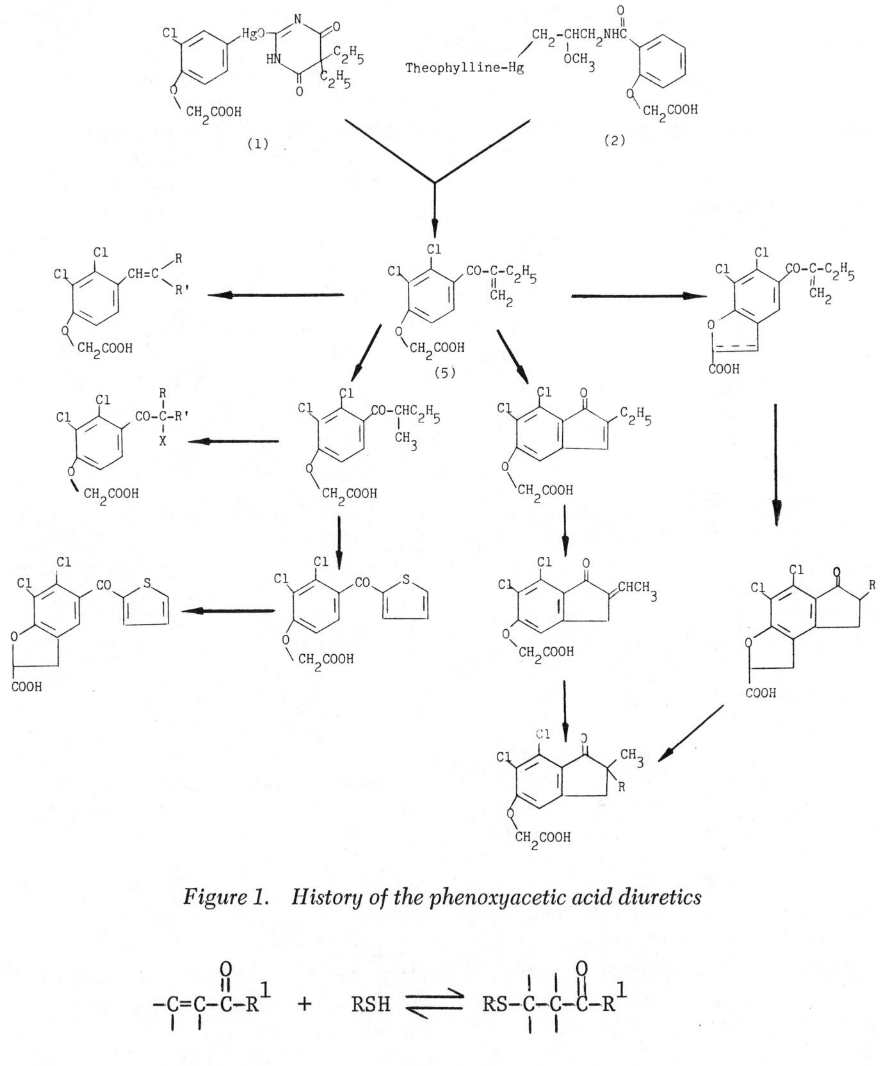

Figure 1. History of the phenoxyacetic acid diuretics

$$-\underset{|}{\overset{|}{C}}=\underset{|}{\overset{|}{C}}-\overset{O}{\overset{\|}{C}}-R^1 \quad + \quad RSH \quad \rightleftharpoons \quad RS-\underset{|}{\overset{|}{C}}-\underset{|}{\overset{|}{C}}-\overset{O}{\overset{\|}{C}}-R^1$$

(3)

$$H-Hg-R^2 \quad + \quad RSH \quad \rightleftharpoons \quad R-S-Hg-R^2$$

(4)

Figure 2. Reaction of α,β-unsaturated ketones and mercurials with mercaptans

was disappointing, but a knowledge of the critical structural
requirements of the organic moiety for mercurials led us to
prepare an organic portion of the α,β-unsaturated ketones more
akin to that of merbaphen. This was achieved in compound 4
which, to our delight, had diuretic properties. The activity
was very weak and of short duration, but it had the qualitative
properties we were seeking. Thus, a lead had been established
which, upon development, ultimately led to the discovery of
ethacrynic acid (Compound 5, Figure 1) (4).

(3)   (4)

The information generated by the research in the ethacrynic
acid series set off an explosion of ideas on the design of new
diuretics both in our laboratories and in others. The history of
how this family of diuretics evolved is illustrated graphically
in Figure 1. The arrows portray the geneological relationship
of each member of the family which will be discussed system-
atically in this paper. Interestingly, many of these structural
types exhibit qualitatively and quantitatively different renal
characteristics.

(Acryloylphenoxy)acetic Acids - After having established compound 4 as a lead, its development involved a systematic structural variation and correlation of biological activity with a
series of physical properties, including pKa, H_2O/lipid distribution, protein binding, etc. In addition, correlation of some
chemical properties was investigated. The compounds were
initially screened intravenously in dogs where the sodium,
potassium and chloride excretion and urine volumes were measured
in comparison to controls. For convenience, the compounds were
scored according to the criterion in Table I.
    We first investigated the optimum location of the oxyacetic
acid group in relation to the substituted acryloyl moiety of
compound 4 (Table II). When these groups were ortho to each
other, the compound was inactive. With the meta-orientation,
activity was improved, but the para-orientation was optimal.
    Next, attention was focused on the role of nuclear sub-
stituents (Table III). Only marginal activity was seen when the
four nuclear substituents were hydrogen, and substituents in the
2-position made little contribution to activity. In the 3-
position, although fluoro had little effect, the other halo,
methyl and trifluoromethyl substituents bestowed a marked increase on the activity. The combined effect of two chloro

TABLE I

Scoring System

Dog Assay[a]

5 mg/kg i.v. Stat Dose

Score	μEq. Na$^+$/Min. Excreted
0	0 - 99
±	Active Above 5 mg/kg
1	100 - 399
2	400 - 599
3	600 - 799
4	800 - 899
5	900 - 999
6	>1000

[a]Female animals were starved overnight, anesthetized with phenobarbital, creatinine primed, catheterized and infused with phosphate buffer at a rate of 3 ml/min. The drug was given i.v. at 5 mg/kg over a period of 5 min, and 15-min collections of urine were taken over a period of 2 h. The data recorded were the average of the two highest consecutive 15-min collections.

TABLE II

Effect of Location of the Acryloyl Moiety

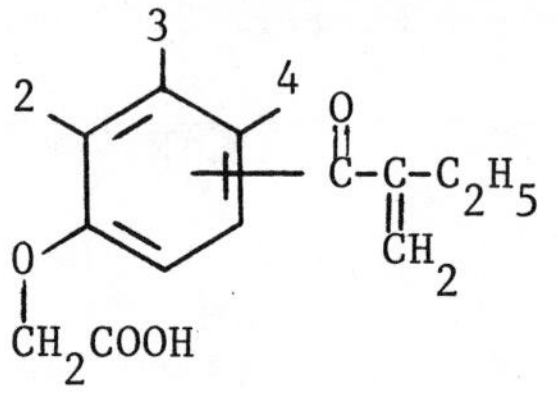

Ring Position of $C_2H_5-\underset{\underset{CH_2}{\|}}{C}-\underset{\underset{O}{\|}}{C}-$	Cl	I.V. Dog Na$^+$ Scores
2	4	$\pm$
3	4	2
4	3	4

TABLE III

Effect of Nuclear Substituents

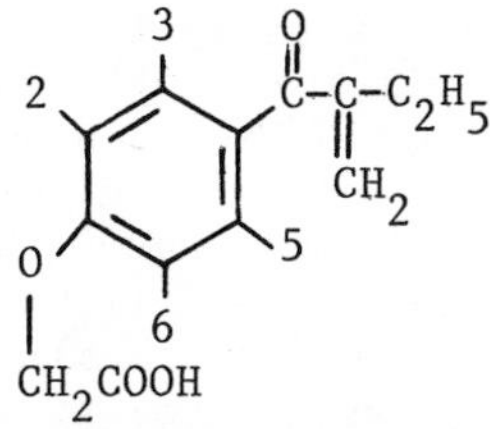

$$\underset{CH_2COOH}{\overset{O}{\underset{5}{\overset{3}{\underset{6}{\overset{2}{\bigcirc}}}}}} \overset{O}{\underset{CH_2}{\overset{\|}{C}}}-C-C_2H_5$$

	Substituents				I.V. Dog Na$^+$ Score	T$_{1/2}^a$
	2	3	5	6		
	H	H	H	H	±	>90
(MK-495)	Cl	H	H	H	±	27
	CH$_3$	H	H	H	0	>90
	H	F	H	H	±	27
	H	Cl	H	H	4	7
	H	Br	H	H	4	9
	H	I	H	H	4	9
	H	CF$_3$	H	H	3	14
	H	CH$_3$	H	H	3	48
	H	C$_2$H$_5$	H	H	±	43
(MK-595)	Cl	Cl	H	H	6	6
	Cl	H	Cl	H	±	6
	H	Cl	Cl	H	3	6
	Cl	H	H	Cl	±	22
(MK-695)	CH$_3$	CH$_3$	H	H	5	45
	CH$_3$	H	CH$_3$	H	0	58
	CH$_3$	H	H	CH$_3$	0	165
	CH$_3$	CH$_3$	CH$_3$	H	±	75
	CH$_3$	CH$_3$	H	CH$_3$	±	73
	CH$_3$	CH$_3$	CH$_3$	CH$_3$	±	60

^{a}Time in minutes required for 50% reaction with a standard solution of mercaptoacetic acid.

(MK-595, ethacrynic acid) or two methyl groups (MK-695) located
in the 2- and 3-positions produced a dramatic increase in
diuretic activity. Other orientations of two chloro or methyl
groups were much less effective and each of the trimethyl and
the tetramethyl analogs were virtually inactive.

As we had anticipated, the (acryloylphenoxy)acetic acids
and the mercurial diuretics exhibited marked similarities in
their reaction with sulfhydryl-containing compounds, both in
vitro and in vivo (3, 4, 5). A measure of this property was
recorded for each of our compounds as illustrated in the column
headed $T_{\frac{1}{2}}$, which is actually the time in minutes required for
each compound to give a 50% complete reaction with a standard
concentration of mercaptoacetic acid at pH 7.4. These data
indicate that the most active compounds react very rapidly with
this model sulfhydryl reagent. Although, as one might expect,
some compounds which react rather slowly have fairly good
diuretic activity, and some that react very rapidly are inactive, e.g., the first compound, because they fail to meet
other structural or chemical requirements. Compounds containing
5- and 6-substituents were markedly less active. This led us to
believe that either the 2- and 3-positions (or the 5- and
6-positions) must remain unsubstituted to maintain activity. As
will be seen later, this idea was dramatically disproved in two
instances.

A few of the compounds that were prepared to evaluate the
effect of substituents on the vinyl carbon atoms appear in Table
IV. The first compound (where each R=H) reacts so rapidly and
irreversibly with many nucleophiles (in contradistinction to the
other compounds in this series) that it possesses very little
activity. Each of the compounds bearing a single alpha (R^1)
substituent, whether alkyl or cycloalkyl, exhibited potent
diuretic activity and a rapid reaction with mercaptoacetic acid.
The detrimental effect of an alkyl substituent on both the alpha
(R^1) and the beta (R^2) carbon atom was even more pronounced when
alkyl groups occupied both beta (R^2 and R^3) atoms. Hydroxy and
methoxy groups on the beta (R^2) carbon atom were not tolerated.

Several compounds were studied in which the ether oxygen
atom was replaced by other functionalities (Table V). Replacement of oxygen by sulfur provided compounds that were as potent
as their oxygen isosteres; however, the corresponding sulfoxides
possessed little activity. Replacement of oxygen by -NH-,
-N(CH$_3$)- or -CH$_2$- drastically reduced or abolished activity.
However, replacement of the oxygen atom by a bond provided the
corresponding phenylacetic acids which possessed modest activity.

Representatives of the many groups which were evaluated as
surrogates for the carboxymethyl moiety (R) are listed in Table
VI. When a methylene proton is replaced by fluoro, full activity is maintained. However, substitution of one methylene
proton by a methyl group is detrimental and substitution of both

TABLE IV

Effect of Substituents on the Vinyl Carbon Atoms

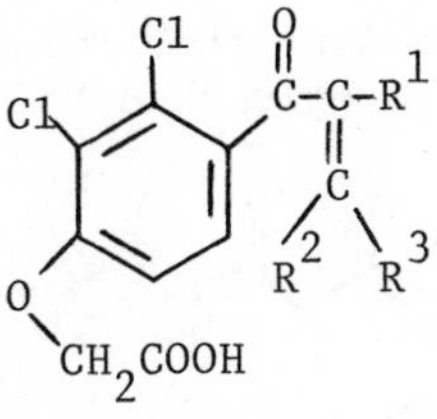

R^1	R^2	R^3	I.V. Dog Na$^+$ Score	$T_{1/2}$
-H	H	H	$\pm$	<1
-CH$_3$	H	H	5	1
-C$_2$H$_5$	H	H	6	6
-CH$_2$(CH$_3$)$_2$	H	H	5	5
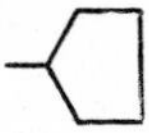 ⬠	H	H	very active[a]	<94
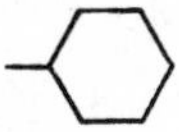 ⬡	H	H	very active[a]	<55
-CH$_3$	CH$_3$	H	2	109
-C$_2$H$_5$	CH$_3$	H	5	>120
-H	CH$_3$	CH$_3$	1	109
-C$_2$H$_5$	OH	H	$\pm$	0
-C$_2$H$_5$	OCH$_3$	H	$\pm$	131

[a]Only tested by p.o. route

TABLE V

Effect of Varying the Atom that Bridges the Nucleus
with the Acetic Acid Moiety

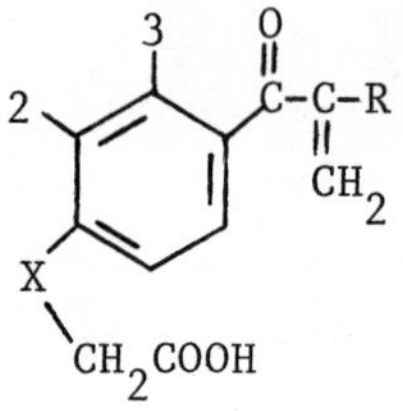

X	2	3	R	I.V. Dog Na$^+$ Score
-O-	H	Cl	CH_3	3
-O-	Cl	Cl	C_2H_5	6
-S-	H	Cl	CH_3	3
-S-	Cl	Cl	C_2H_5	6
-SO-	Cl	Cl	C_2H_5	$\pm$
-NH-	H	Cl	CH_3	$\pm$
-NCH$_3$-	H	Cl	CH_3	0
-CH$_2$-	H	Cl	CH_3	0
-	H	Cl	C_2H_5	2

TABLE VI

Effect of Varying the Oxyacetic Acid Group

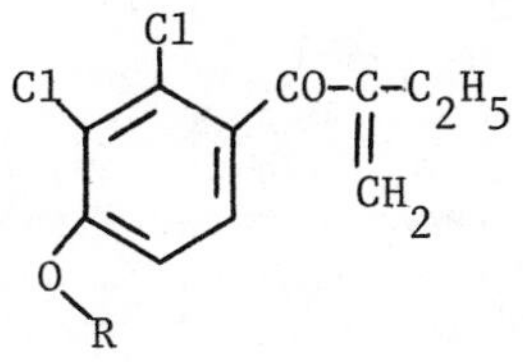

R	I.V. Dog Na^+ Score	$T_{1/2}$
$-CHFCOOH$	6	–
$-CH(CH_3)COOH$	2	2
$-C(CH_3)_2COOH$	±	<1
$-(CH_2)_3COOH$	1	<17
$-H$	±	<26
$-CH_2CONH_2$	±	6
$-CH_2COOC_2H_5$	very active[a]	12
$-CH_2SO_3^- Na^+$	6	<4
$-SO_2N(CH_3)_2$	active[a]	–

[a]Tested orally

of them by methyl groups is disastrous, as is lengthening the
chain by two methylene units. The phenol (R=H) and the acetamide
(R=CH$_2$CONH$_2$) have little activity, but the ethyl ester is fully
active. Replacement of carboxy by sulfonate (R=CH$_2$SO$_3$Na) gives a
compound which is highly active i.v. but not p.o. Interestingly,
the compound where R=SO$_2$N(CH$_3$)$_2$ exhibits oral activity.

The structure/activity (S/A) data on the (acryloylphenoxy)-
acetic acids which we have presented indicate that both substitution of the 6-position of the nucleus and introduction of a
methyl group on the carbon atom alpha to carboxy have detrimental effects on activity. However, a number of patents (e.g.,
7, 8) have been assigned to Ciba-Geigy on benzofurans that can be
viewed as 6 to α-cyclization products (Table VII) which violate
both of these S/A indications. We prepared some examples of these
structures, including the two shown in Table VII, and found them
to be active in dogs, but the saturated forms were more active
than the aromatic analogs (in which the double bond is present).
It should be noted that these compounds have 6,7-dimethyl substituents and that the analogous (acryloylphenoxy)acidic acids
are less active than the corresponding dichloro compounds (see
Table III).

Many studies on the site and mode of action of ethacrynic
acid have been reported. This compound belongs to the class of
potent"loop" diuretics, which includes furosemide and bumetanide,
since its principle action is in the distal portion of the loop of
Henle (9-13). Like the mercurial diuretics (6), ethacrynic acid
is excreted partially as the cysteine adduct (5) which has been
shown to be active in man (14). The mercurials and ethacrynic
acid also show similar effects on decreasing the protein-bound
sulfhydryl groups in renal cells in dogs. No such effect was
observed in rats, a species in which the drug is virtually inactive (15-18).

Ethacrynic acid and its analogs are readily cyclized to the
corresponding indanones (I), shown in Table VIII, which can be
brominated (II) and selectively dehydrobrominated to the corresponding indenones (III) or 2-alkylideneindanones (IV). Although
Topliss (19) had found a deschloro analog to be inactive, compounds bearing chlorine atoms in the 6- and 7-positions were
highly active, as seen with the two compounds listed on the second
line of Table VIII which are the precise analogs of ethacrynic
acid. This constitutes the second exception to the idea that the
5- and 6-positions must remain unsubstituted. Branching (i.e.,
where R and R^1 are CH$_3$) decreases activity in both series.

A hypothesis regarding the behavior of the (acryloylphenoxy)acetic acids (V) in body fluids is illustrated in Figure
3 which shows their reaction with a variety of sulfhydryl-
containing compounds (VI), particularly cysteine and glutathione, to form adducts (VII). Upon reaching the nephron, a
reaction occurs with the receptor sulfhydryl group (R SH, VIII)

TABLE VII

Benzofuran Analogs of (Acryloylphenoxy)acetic Acids

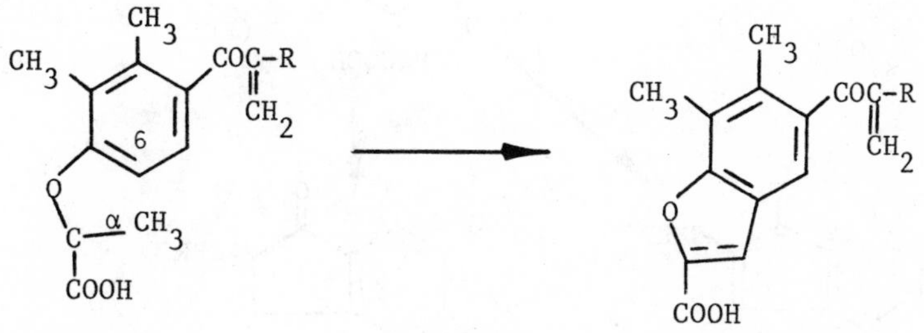

R	Double Bond Present	I.V. Dog Na^+ Score
$-CH(CH_3)_2$	NO	3
$-(CH_2)_2CH_3$	YES	1

TABLE VIII

Cyclic Analogs of (Acryloylphenoxy)acetic Acids

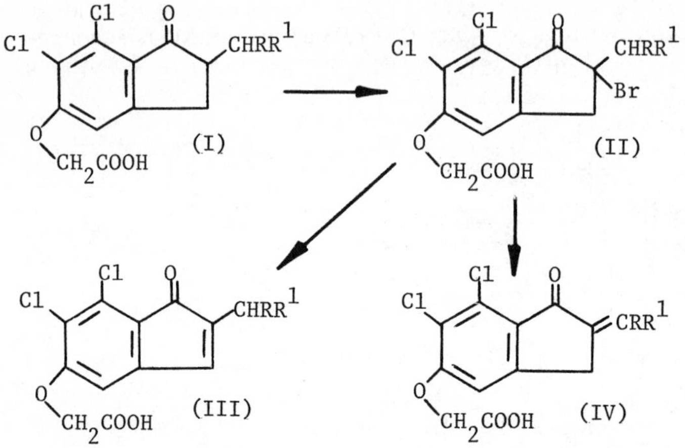

| R | R^1 | I.V. Dog Na$^+$ Scores | |
		Indenyloxyacetic Acid (III)	2-Alkylidene-indanyloxyacetic Acid (IV)
H	H	4	–
CH$_3$	H	4	4
CH$_3$	CH$_3$	3	2
-(CH$_2$)-		–	1
Ethacrynic Acid		6	–

to give a new adduct (IX). For each compound, the diuretic
activity will depend, in part, on the equilibrium constants for
reaction 1 vs. reaction 2 and the reaction rates. The most
active compounds will be those whose equilibrium constants and
reaction rates favor the receptor adducts (IX).

Confirmation of this concept was attempted by preparing
some mercaptan adducts of ethacrynic acid and studying their
diuretic effects in dogs (Table IX). It is seen that the methyl
mercaptan adduct has only weak activity, but that the corresponding sulfoxide and sulfone are about as active as ethacrynic
acid. From these selected examples, it will be seen that a
range of activities are obtained, from that as great as ethacrynic acid, i.e., the cysteine and glutathione adducts, to
complete inactivity, i.e., the mercaptoacetic and N-acetyl-
cysteine adducts.

In the ethacrynic acid series, Free-Wilson and similar
analysis were found to be of little value. However, a study by
G. B. Smith and G. V. Downing proved to be quite enlightening.
They prepared the contour map shown in Figure 4 which shows the
correlation of each compound's distribution coefficient (between
chloroform and pH 7.4 buffer) with its rate constant for reaction with mercaptoacetic acid. Each point shown on the map
represents one compound with its i.v. dog diuretic score beneath
the point. When either distribution coefficients or rate
constants are considered separately, no correlation is evident;
however, when both parameters are considered and lines drawn
connecting points of equal diuretic activity, order emerges.
The map defines regions or island of each activity which provided guidance in the design of compounds with maximal activity.

[4-(2-Haloacyl)phenoxy]acetic Acids - Another class of potent
diuretics are those of the type shown in Table X. The most
active members are those where R is alkyl or cycloalkyl, R^1=H
and X=bromo. Comparing those where R=isopropyl, the compound in
which X=Br is superior to those where X=Cl or I. These compounds react with mercaptans, but some of the most diuretic
members react very slowly and the products of the reaction are
different from those obtained with the acryloylphenoxyacetic
acids, i.e., the X is replaced by H, while the mercaptan is
oxidized to the disulfide.

(Vinylaryloxy)acetic Acids - About the time that the S/A relationships in the (acryloylphenoxy)acetic acid series seemed
clear, compound 2 (Table XI) was prepared in which the carbonyl
and vinyl groups were interchanged ([20]). The unexpected activity of this compound suggested the synthesis of the lower
homolog (Compound 1) which was more active, and the introduction
of a methyl group at R^1 which increased the activity (Compound
3). The introduction of a methyl at R^1 on compound 2 markedly
decreased the activity (compound 4), but the cyclization to the

TABLE IX

Mercaptan Adducts of Ethacrynic Acid

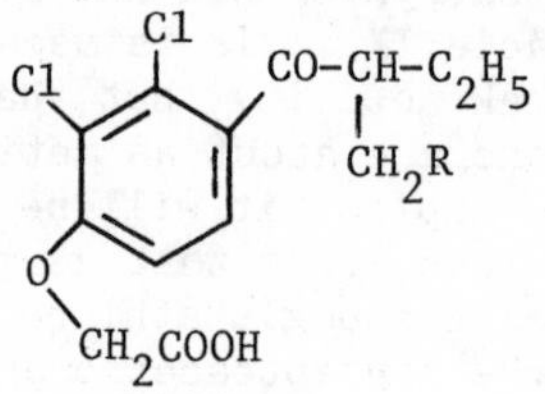

R	I.V. Dog Na^+ Score	R	I.V. Dog Na^+ Score
$-SCH_3$	2	$-SCH_2COOH$	0
$-SOCH_3$	6	$-SCH_2CH(NHCOCH_3)COOH$	$\pm$
$-SO_2CH_3$	5	$-SCH_2CH(NH_2)COOH$	6
$-SCH_2-$	3	$-SG$ (glutathione)	6.
$-SC(CH_3)_3$	2	$-SCOCH_3$	4
$-S(CH_2)_4Cl$	1	$-S)_2$	2
$-S-$	$\pm$	$-SO_3^-Na^+$	0

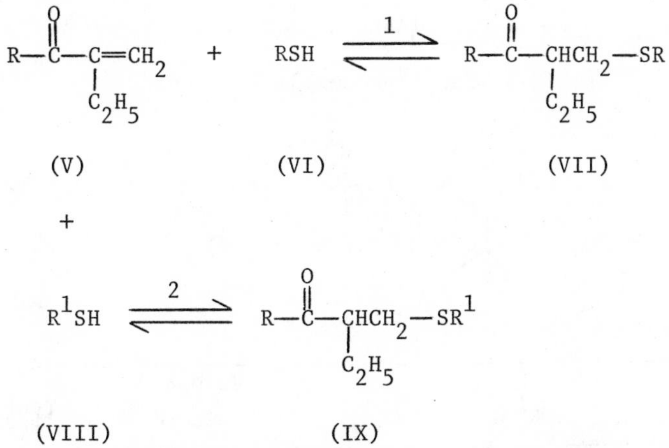

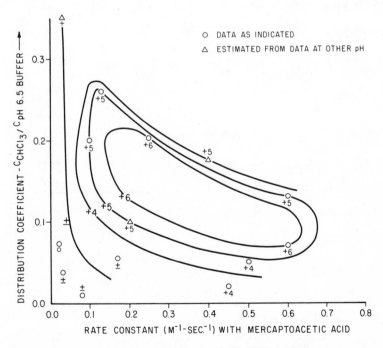

Figure 3. *Reaction of (acryloylphenoxy)acetic acids with sulfhydryl compounds*

Figure 4. *Activity contour map—chloroform distribution vs. rate constant*

TABLE X

[4-(2-Haloacyl)phenoxy]acetic Acids

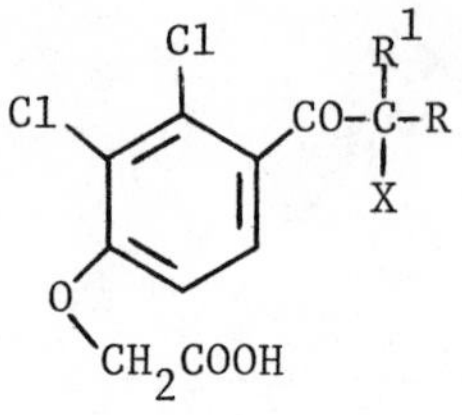

R	R^1	X	I.V. Dog Na$^+$ Score	$T_{1/2}$
$-C_2H_5$	H	Br	5	21
$-CH(CH_3)_2$	H	Cl	$\pm$	No R_x
$-CH(CH_3)_2$	H	Br	5	41
$-CH(CH_3)_2$	H	I	2	
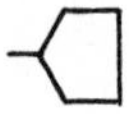 ⬠	H	Br	6	>120
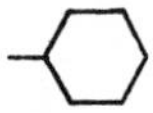 ⬡	H	Br	very active[a]	
$-C_2H_5$	CH_3	Br	+	21
$-C_2H_5$	C_2H_5	Br	$\pm$	41

[a]Active orally

TABLE XI

(Vinylphenoxy)acetic Acids

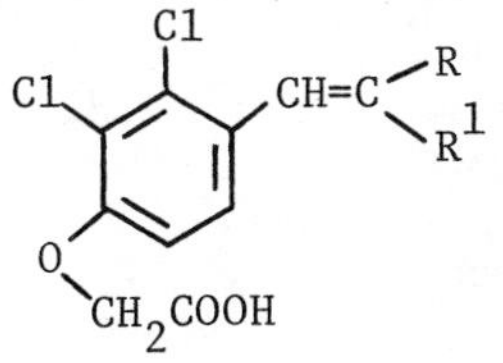

Compound	R	R^1	I.V. Dog Na^+ Score	$T_{1/2}$
1	CH_3CO-	$H-$	5	56
2	C_2H_5CO-	$H-$	4	No Rx
3	CH_3CO-	CH_3-	6	
4	C_2H_5CO-	CH_3-	±	No Rx
5	$-COCH_2CH_2CH-$		6*	Very Slow
6	CH_3CO-	CH_3CO-	6*	2
7	CH_3CO	C_2H_5CO-	6*	2
8	C_2H_5CO-	C_2H_5CO-	4*	5
9	NO_2-	$H-$	1*	<1
10	NO_2-	CH_3-	6*	<1
11	NO_2-	C_2H_5-	6*	2
12	NO_2-	$CH_3(CH_2)_4-$	3*	8
13	$CN-$	$H-$	4*	No Rx
14	C_2H_5OOC-	C_2H_5OOC-	1	13
15	H_2NCO-	H_2NCO-	±	79
16	$-COCH(CH_2CH_2)_2N-$		3*	Very Slow

*Estimated from the response at a dose below 5 mg/kg

corresponding cyclopentanone (Compound 5) greatly increased
activity.

Extending the series (21) to those where both R and R^1 are
acyl groups greatly enhanced the activity with maximal potency
appearing when both groups are acetyl (Compound 6). The compounds where R represents NO_2 (22) also were very active.
Increased potency was observed when the second group (R^1) was
methyl or ethyl (Compounds 10 and 11). Similar but weaker
activity was observed in a number of other compounds (23) in
which R and R^1 represent a variety of electron-withdrawing
groups, i.e., cyano, ethoxycarbonyl, carbamoyl and sulfamoyl.
The most active compounds, i.e., compounds 6-11, react the most
avidly with mercaptoacetic acid.

In each series, the other structural requirements for
activity paralleled that found for the (acryloylphenoxy)acetic
acids. One notable difference was the high activity of
mercaptan adducts which were inactive in the (acryloylphenoxy)-
acetic acid series. Thus, compound 6 and its mercaptoacetic
acid adduct were equipotent, while the corresponding adduct of
ethacrynic acid was inactive.

Oral studies (Table XII) in dogs on representatives from
each series indicate that compound 3 is four times as potent as
furosemide, compound 6 is 70 times and compound 10 is 30 times
as active.

We have discussed the three general types of phenoxyacetic
acids shown in Figure 5. They each can react with sulfhydryl
compounds, but each involves a different site on the molecule as
shown by the arrows. Our current concept is that, although
these compounds can react with receptor sulfhydryl groups and
that such a reaction contributes to their activity, this reaction is not critical for saluresis. A series of (2,3-dichloro-
4-saturated-acylphenoxy)acetic acids, which cannot react with
sulfhydryl groups, were made and tested in dogs (Table XIII).
Many of these exhibited appreciable saluresis. Particularly
significant are dihydroethacrynic acid (Compound 1) and the
water adduct of ethacrynic acid (Compound 4) which exhibited
weak, but significant activity. Although these compounds exhibited only modest activity, this observation was of profound
theoretical significance and set the stage for a major breakthrough in the (acylphenoxy)acetic acid family of diuretics. To
obtain a complete picture, the compounds that were made for
subsequent studies were evaluated orally in chimpanzees, rats
and dogs according to the criterion shown in Tables XIV, XV and
XVI.

Evaluation of "dihydroethacrynic acid" (Compound 1, Table
XIII) in chimpanzees revealed that it had a weak but significant
saluretic activity and that, in contrast to ethacrynic acid, it
was uricosuric.

(1-Oxoindanyloxy)acetic Acids - Since 2-halo compounds,
such as compound 1 in Table XVII, had been used to synthesize the

TABLE XII

Oral Dog Activity of (Vinylphenoxy)acetic Acids

Cmpd. No. from Table XI	mg/kg p.o. Dose	Ave. 6 hr. mEq. Excretion[a]		
		Na^+	K^+	Cl^-
3	2	16	3	21
6	0.4	34	6	36
10	0.4	23	6	29
11	1	24	5	26
16	5	12	4	17
Furosemide	0.4	8	3	11
	10	19	4	18
Placebo	–	2	1	2

[a] Oral tests were carried out on a colony of trained female mongrel dogs weighing 8–10 kg. All dogs received 100 ml of water the previous day and were fasted overnight. On the day of the test, 250 ml of water was administered orally, followed by 500 ml of water (orally) 1 hr later. One hour after the last oral priming dose of water, bladders were emptied by catheterization and the study was commenced by administration of compound or placebo. Compounds were given in gelatin capsules and the animals were maintained in metabolism cages for collection of spontaneously voided urine. Spontaneous urine was combined with bladder urine collected by catheterization at the end of 6 hr. Urine volumes were measured, and aliquots were analyzed for sodium, potassium and chloride content by standard methodology. Values are reported as geometric means.

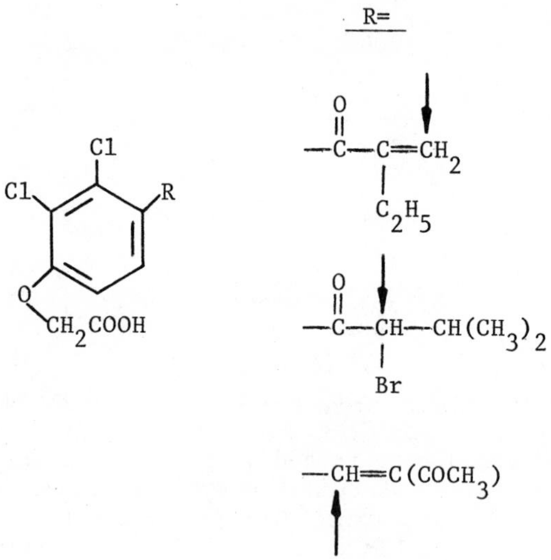

Figure 5. Site of reaction

TABLE XIII

(2,3-Dichloro-4-saturated-acylphenoxy)acetic Acids

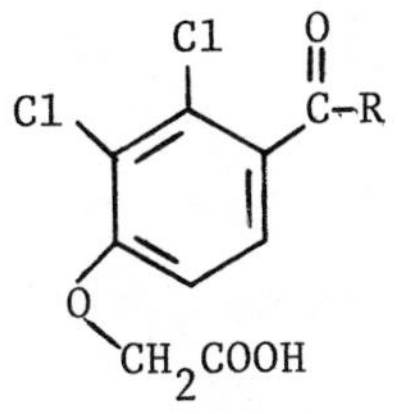

Compd. No.	R	I.V. Dog Na$^+$ Score
1	$-CH(CH_3C_2H_5$	2*
2	$-CH_2C_2H_5$	1
3	$-C(C_2H_5)-OCH_2$	3
4	$-CH(CH_2OH)C_2H_5$	3
5	$-CH(CH_2CN)C_2H_5$	2
Ethacrynic Acid		6

*Estimated value from data at 1 mg/kg

TABLE XIV

Chimpanzee Data: Excretion following
0.5 mg/kg i.v. or 5 mg/kg p.o.[a]

μEq/Min Na$^+$	Score	Δ^{C}Urate/^{C}Inulin
0-49	0	0-.05
50-99	$\pm$	.05-.09
100-199	1	.10-.19
200-299	2	.20-.29
300-399	3	.30-.39
400-499	4	.40-.49
500 and Above	5	.50 and Above

[a]Fasted, male chimpanzees weighing 21-77 kg were immobilized
with phencyclidine (which was shown not to affect the results)
(1.0-1.5 mg/kg i.m. plus 0.25 mg/kg i.v. as needed) and were
prepared by catheterization for standard renal clearance
studies using routine clinical asceptic procedures. Pyrogen-
free inulin (i.v.) was used to measure glomeruluar filtration
rate (GFR). Clearance of inulin, urate and the excretion
rates of Na$^+$, K$^+$ and Cl$^-$ were determined by standard Auto
Analyzer techniques. (Inulin and urate in chimpanzee plasma
are freely filterable.) Average control clearances were
calculated from three 20-min consecutive periods. Drug-
response values were derived as the average of eight 15-
20 min clearance periods after oral administration of an
aqueous solution of the compound through an indwelling nasal
catheter. All data are reported as the difference between
(average) treatment and control values obtained from single
experiments.

TABLE XV

5 Hr. p.o. Rat Scoring System[a]

Score	mEquivalents of Na^+ at the Given mg/kg Dose				
	0	3	9	27	81
0	.3	.3	.3	.3	.3
±	.3	.3	.3	.5	.9
1	.3	.3	.4	.7	1.5
2	.3	.3	.5	1.1	2.4
3	.3	.3	.9	1.9	2.9
4	.3	1.0	2.1	2.9	–
5	.3	1.7	2.9	3.4	–
6	.3	2.9	3.9	4.1	–

[a]Female rats (Charles River, 150–170 g) were maintained over-night on a sugar diet with water ad libitum. The test substance was dissolved in pure DMF and subsequently diluted with water (which contained 3 drops of Tween-80 per 100 ml) such that the final vehicle was 4% DMF. At the time of the test, animals were given the vehicle (as placebo) or test substance suspended in a final volume of 5.0 ml p.o. Rats were housed in groups of three in metabolism cages. Urine was collected for the 0–5 hr interval in graduated cylinders and was analyzed for sodium, potassium and chloride content. Animals that received placebo were run concurrently. Results are reported as milliequivalents per cage and are the geometric means of three cages per dose level. Standard methodology was used for determination of electrolyte levels.

TABLE XVI

5 Hr. p.o. Dog Scoring System[a]

| Score | mEquivalents of Na^+ at the Given mg/kg Dose | | | | | |
	0	1	2	5	10	20
0	2	2	2	2	2	2
±	2	2	2	2	8	>8
1	2	2	2	8	15	25
2	2	2	8	15	25	35
3	2	8	15	25	35	45
4	2	15	25	35	45	55
5	2	25	35	45	55	65

[a]Oral tests were carried out on a colony of trained female mongrel dogs weighing 8–10 kg. All dogs received 100 ml of water the previous day and were fasted overnight. On the day of the test, 250 ml of water was administered orally, followed by 500 ml of water (orally) 1 hr later. One hour after the last oral priming dose of water, bladders were emptied by catheterization and the study was commenced by administration of compound or placebo. Compounds were given in gelatin capsules and the animals were maintained in metabolism cages for collection of spontaneously voided urine. Spontaneous urine was combined with bladder urine collected by catheterization at the end of 5 hr. Urine volumes were measured, and aliquots were analyzed for sodium, potassium and chloride content by standard methodology. Values are reported as geometric means.

TABLE XVII

2-Substituted-Indanones

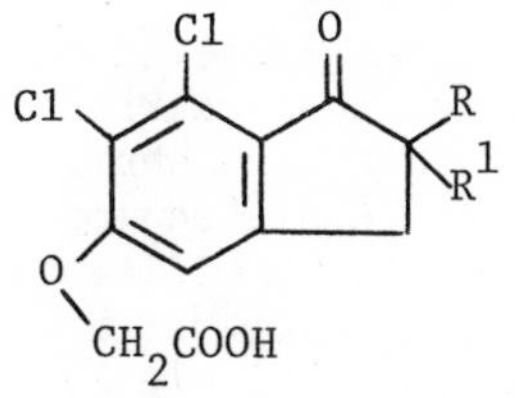

Compd No.	R	R^1	P.O. Na^+ Score Rat	P.O. Na^+ Score Dog	P.O. Chimp Score Na^+	P.O. Chimp Score Urate
1	$-C_2H_5$	-Cl	3	1	2	±
2	-H	-H	0	0		
3	$-CH_3$	-H	2	1		
4	-Et	-H	2	1	4	±
5	-Pr	-H	±	1	5	1
6	-i-Pr	-H	2	3	5	2
7	-Bu	-H	±	1	1	1
8	-sec-Bu	-H	2	±		
9	-t-Bu	-H	2	2	1	±
10	-Am	-H	1	1	1	±
11		-H	1	1	5	2
12		-H	1	1	2	3
13		-H	1		3	1
	Ethacrynic Acid		0	6	5	0 (retains urate)

(indenyloxy)acetic acids and the (2-alkylideneindanyloxy)acetic
acids described in Table VIII, the possibility that it could
function as a pro-drug was considered. However, its saluretic
activity in rats and its uricosuric activity in chimpanzees
revealed it to be qualitatively distinct from the mercurials and
the unsaturated aryloxyacetic acids. It was assumed that the
observed biological differences were due to the unchanged
compound, even though metabolic studies indicated that some of
the expected dehydrohalogenation had occurred. This led us to
prepare analogs of compound 1 that were chemically more stable,
such as compound 4, which is an annulated form of "dihydroethacrynic acid" (24-27). Its activity profile was very similar to
that of compound 1.

The representative compounds of Table XVII exhibit a range
of saluretic and uricosuric responses when R represents a
variety of alkyl, cycloalkyl and aryl substituents. The 2-
isopropyl analog (Compound 6) appeared to have the overall
optimum activity. The effect of structural modification of the
nuclear substituents and reorientation or variation of the
oxyacetic acid moiety was about the same as had been observed in
the (aryloxy)acetic acid series.

A most significant contribution to the activity of these
(indanyloxy)acetic acids (27-28) occurred with the introduction
of a second 2-substituent (Table XVIII). These compounds were
generally considerably more active than the corresponding
monosubstituted compounds. To quantitate these comparisons in
rats, dose-response curves with high statistical significance
were developed. The numbers in parenthesis in Table XVIII are
the fold greater activity found for each 2-R, 2-CH$_3$ compound as
compared to the monosubstituted analog (Compound 1). Optimal
diuretic activity was seen with compounds 4 and 6 (MK-196), but
the latter compound exhibited optimal dual (diuretic-uricosuric)
activity. Increasing the size of R to ethyl (Compounds 7 and 8)
was detrimental to diuretic activity. Since uricosuric and
diuretic activities do not run parallel, some compounds which
are very weak diuretics, e.g., (2-ethyl-3-phenyl-6,7-dichloro-
5-indanyloxy)acetic acid, exhibit potent uricosuric activity.

Substitution on the phenyl group of MK-196 had a marked
effect on diuretic and uricosuric activity (Table XIX). Although
there was considerable species variation, the p-fluoro derivative (Compound 4) showed the best overall activity. Replacement
of the phenyl group of MK-196 by a 2-thienyl group gave a
compound which was equipotent to MK-196. Replacement of the
carboxy group of MK-196 by a number of groups, including 5-
tetrazolyl, usually produced compounds with considerably decreased saluretic activity.

Numerous structural variations were made in positions 1, 2
and 3 of the indane ring (29). Reduction of the 1-oxo group of
MK-196 to hydroxy provided two diasteriomers, both of which were

TABLE XVIII

(2,2-Disubstituted—Indanyloxy)acetic Acids

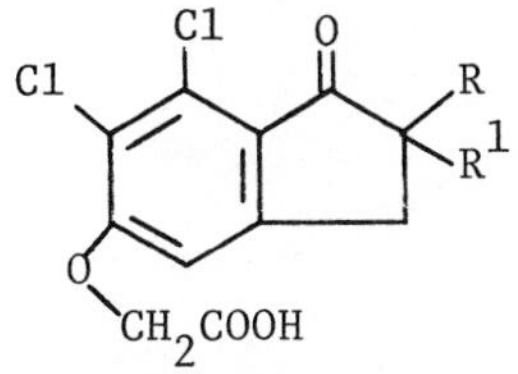

Compd. No.	R	R^1	P.O. Na^+ Scores			P.O. Na^+ Chimp Scores	
			Rat	(FOLD x Compd. 1)	Dog	Na^+	Urate
1	-CH$_3$	H-	2	(1)	1		
2	-CH$_3$	CH$_3$-	3	(4)	1	3	±
3	-Et	CH$_3$-	3	(15)	3	5	1
4	i-Pr	CH$_3$-	3	(53)	3	4	±
5	⊲▢	CH$_3$-	2	(5)	2	2	1
6	⊲⬡	CH$_3$-		(50)	3	5	3
7	⊲▢	C$_2$H$_5$-	2			2	1
8	⊲⬡	C$_2$H$_5$-	1		±	3	1
9	-CH$_2$CH$_2$CH$_2$CH$_2$-		2		1	3	1

TABLE XIX

Effect of Substituents on the Phenyl Group of MK-196

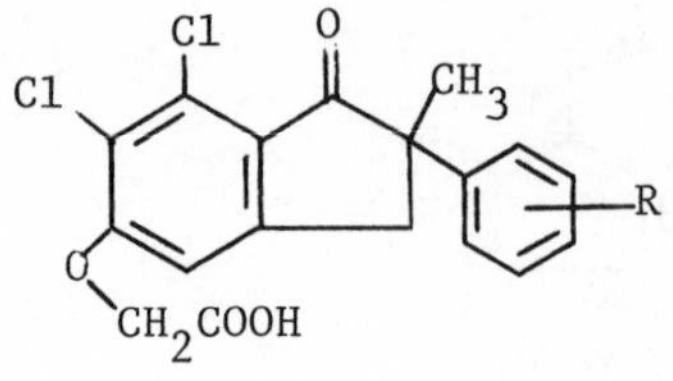

Compd. No.	R	P.O. Na^+ Scores Rat	Dog	P.O. Na^+ Chimp Scores	Urate
1	H	3	3	5	3
2	4-Br	±	1	±	±
3	4-Cl	±	1	3	2
4	4-F	2	3	3	4
5	4-OCH_3	2		4	±
6	4-OH	±	2	1	±
7	3-OH	1	2		
8	4-NH_2	1	1	2	±
9	4-NO_2	4	2	1	±
10	4-SO_2NH_2	1	5	5	±
11	4-$COCH_3$	±		5	±

about as active as the parent (30). Alkyl or aryl groups in the
3-position usually decreased saluretic activity, and either did
not affect or increased the uricosuric activity. A 3-oxo substituent generally provided compounds with activities only
slightly below that of their parents (31).

The influence of the chiral center at the 2-position can be
seen from the study involving the four enantiomeric pairs (Table
XX). Although there was some variation among species, the
enantiomeric effect was most pronounced with compounds 1 and 4.

Four of the (indanyloxy)acetic acids have been studied
clinically: compounds 6 and 11 from Table XVII and compounds 5
(MK-473) and 8 (MK-196) from Table XVIII. The relative saluretic
and uricosuric potencies in man were predictable from the animal
data, i.e., MK-196>MK-473>compound 11>compound 6 (Table XVII).

MK-196 has received extensive pharmacological, biochemical
and clinical evaluation (32-34). It produced a sustained antihypertensive effect in SH rats (32-33) at oral doses of 0.5-7.5
mg/kg. It was more potent than furosemide or hydrochlorothiazide
when given daily for three days. It also was antihypertensive in
renal hypertensive monkeys but not in renal hypertensive dogs.

MK-196 is well absorbed in mice, rats, dogs, monkeys,
chimpanzees and humans (34-36). In rats and dogs, there was
little metabolism of the drug, which is excreted mainly in the
feces. In mice and monkeys, there was some metabolism and about
equal elimination by the fecal and urinary routes. In chimpanzees, the major elimination is via the urine and, in man there is
considerable metabolism, primarily to the 2-(p-hydroxyphenyl)
derivative (Compound 6, Table XIX).

In chimpanzees (37-39), the urinary excretion of MK-196 is
increased ten-fold when the urine is alkaline. The drug is secreted by the renal tubule and passively back-diffuses across the
tubular epithelium by a pH-dependent process.

Since it is known that urate is reabsorbed and secreted in
the proximal tubule, the studies in chimpanzees (38) suggested
that the action of MK-196 on the clearance of urate is localized
at this site. Micropuncture studies in rats (40) indicate that
the drug affects electrolyte reabsorption in the loop of Henle
and collecting duct, while concentration gradient studies in
dogs (42) implicate sites in the proximal tubule and ascending
loop of Henle.

Biochemical studies by Kuehl (43) and his colleagues
indicate that MK-196 and other compounds in this series owe at
least part of their activity to their effects on prostaglandin
metabolism. MK-196 and its enantiomers (Table XXI) inhibit
PGE-9-ketoreductase, the enzyme that converts PGE_2 to $PGF_{2\alpha}$. To
a lesser extent, it inhibits PG-15-hydroxydehydrogenase, the
enzyme which deactivates prostaglandins. MK-196 has a greater
inhibitory effect on these enzymes than the classical diuretics
as shown in Table XXI. The overall effect would be to increase
the renal levels of PGE_2.

TABLE XX

Enantiomers of (Indanyloxy)acetic Acids

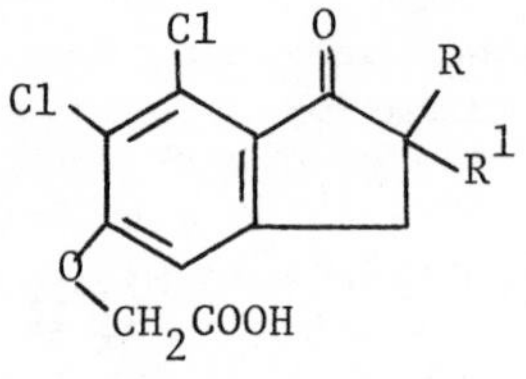

Compd. No.	R	R^1	Enantiomer	P.O. Na$^+$ Scores		P.O. Chimp Scores	
				Rat	Dog	Na$^+$	Urate
1	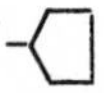 ⬠	H	+	2	2	3	2
			−	1	1	2	1
2	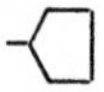 ⬠	CH$_3$	+	3	2	2	1
			−	2	1	2	2
3	-CH(CH$_3$)$_2$	CH$_3$	+	2	3	5	4
			−	3	5	4	1
4	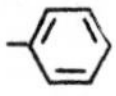 ⬡	CH$_3$	+	1	1	1	1
			−	3	2	6	2
Furosemide				3	5	5	0*
Hydrochlorothiazide				2	2	1	0*
Probenecid							1†

*Decreased Excretion

†Dose = 10 mg/kg

TABLE XXI

Effect of MK-196 on Prostaglandin Metabolism

Compd.	Enantiomer	ID_{50} μM	
		9-Ketoreductase[a]	15-Hydroxydehydrogenase[a]
MK-196	±	15	178
MK-196	+	145	159
MK-196	−	8.5	126
Mersalyl Acid		50	351
Ethacrynic Acid		307	709
Furosemide		499	2419
Hydrochlorothiazide		>2514	>2514

[a]Measured by determining the enzymatic conversion of ^{3}H-PGE$_2$ to [3]H-15-keto-PGE$_2$ in the presence of NADP. [b]Measured by the method of Oien et al (43).

In man, MK-196 (44-46) was found to be a well tolerated saluretic-diuretic. An oral dose of 10 mg elicited a total 24 hour saluresis equivalent to that of 40 mg of furosemide. Administration of furosemide caused a significant increase in plasma urate levels, whereas the continued use of MK-196 caused less increase in plasma urate levels. Daily oral administration of either 10 or 15 mg of MK-196 lowered the blood pressure of hypertensive patients as much as 50 mg of hydrochlorothiazide did. This drug is currently undergoing extensive clinical trials.

Indeno/5,4-b/furan-2-carboxylic Acids - **The interesting activity** exhibited by the benzofuran analogs of the (acryloylphenoxy)- acetic acids of **the type seen in Table VII suggested the** synthesis of some indeno/5,4-b/furan-2-carboxylic acid analogs of the active (indanyloxy)acetic acids. As seen in Table XXII, these compounds are potent diuretics (47, 48). In this series, uricosuric activity was exhibited only by those compounds where R^1 was phenyl. Since these compounds have two chiral centers, two diasteriomers are possible, and in one instance both dia- steriomers (Compounds 3 and 4) were obtained and shown to have quite similar diuretic and uricosuric activities.

(Acylphenoxy)acetic Acids (Table XXIII) - The observation of saluretic and uricosuric activity in tienilic acid (Compound 1, Table XXIII) and some of its analogs (49) and in "dihydro- ethacrynic acid" (Compound 2, Table XXIII) (26) revealed that pharmacodynamic activity existed in several (2,3-dichloro-4- acylphenoxy)acetic acids. The fact that activity also was observed in compound 3 and a number of related structures indicated that the portion of the molecule represented by R could be alkyl, heterocyclic, aryl or aralkyl.

Since annulation of (acryloylphenoxy)acetic acids and (indanyloxy)acetic acids to the corresponding dihydrobenzofurans or dihydroindeno/5,4-b/furans either maintained or improved activity, an analogous annulation of representative (acyl- phenoxy)acetic acids was carried out (50) as recorded in Table XXIV. Studies involving compound 1 in rats, dogs and chimpan- zees revealed it to be 40 to 100 times as potent a diuretic as tienilic acid with about equal activity as a uricosuric agent. Most interesting is the fact that compound 1 is a racemate which upon resolution affords two enantiomers in which there is a complete separation of pharmacodynamic properties. The minus- form possesses only uricosuric activity, while the plus- enantiomer possesses only diuretic properties. This permits the formulation of combinations of the enantiomers to obtain any desired ratio of diuretic to uricosuric activity. It is note- worthy that compounds in which R represents a variety of aryl, aralkyl, or heterocyclic groups retain the activity exhibited by

TABLE XXII

Indeno[5,4-b]Furan-2-Carboxylic Acids

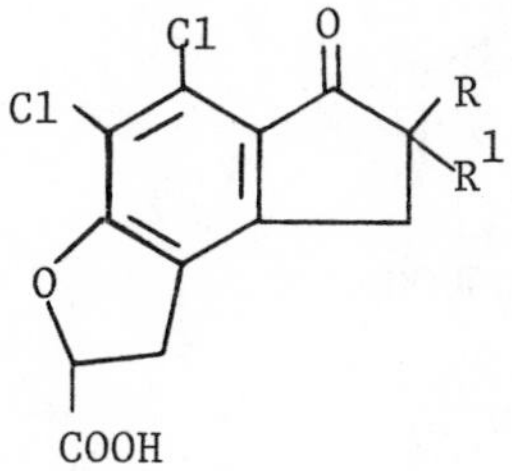

Compd. No.	R	R^1	P.O. Na^+ Scores		P.O. Chimp Scores	
			Rat	Dog	$\frac{P.O.}{Na^+}$	Urate
1	$-(CH_2)_4-$		5	4	5	0
2	CH_3	—▱	4	4	3	0
3 (α)	CH_3	—⬡	3	5	5	5
4 (β)	CH_3	—⬡	4	6	6	4

TABLE XXIII

(4-Acylphenoxy)acetic Acids

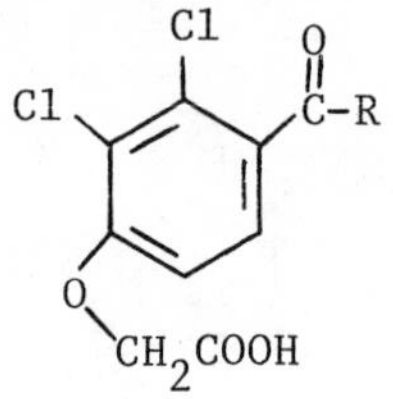

Compd. No.	R	P.O. Rat Scores	I.V. Dog Scores	1 mg/kg I.V. Chimp	
				Na^+ Δ mEq/min	$\dfrac{C_{Urate}}{C_{Inulin}}$
1	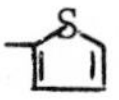 (thiophene ring)	1	1	434	.376
2	$-CH(CH_3)C_2H_5$	$\pm$	1	400	.213
3	$-CH_2-$(phenyl) 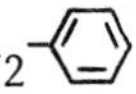	$\pm$	1	363	.309

TABLE XXIV

4-Acyldihydrobenzofurans

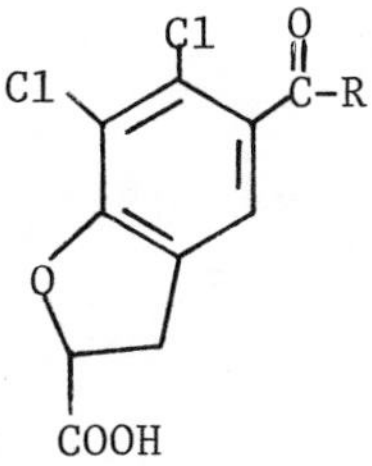

Compd. No.	Enantiomer	R	P.O. Biological Activity Scores			
			Diuretic			Uricosuric Chimp
			Rat	Dog	Chimp	
1	±	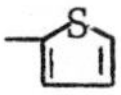	5	4	5	3
	+	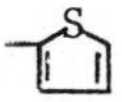	0	0	0	5
	−	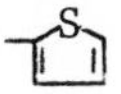	6	5	5	0
2	±	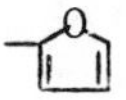	3	3*		
3	±	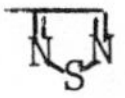	3	3*	5	1
4	±	$-CH_2-$⟨⟩ 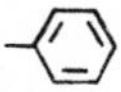	3		4	2
5	±	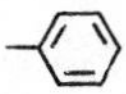 ⟨⟩	3		5	3
6	±	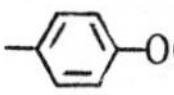 ⟨⟩$-OCH_3$	3			
7	Tienilic Acid		1	±	3	4

*I.V. Scores

TABLE XXV

Reduction Products of 5-Acylbenzofuran-2-Carboxylic Acids

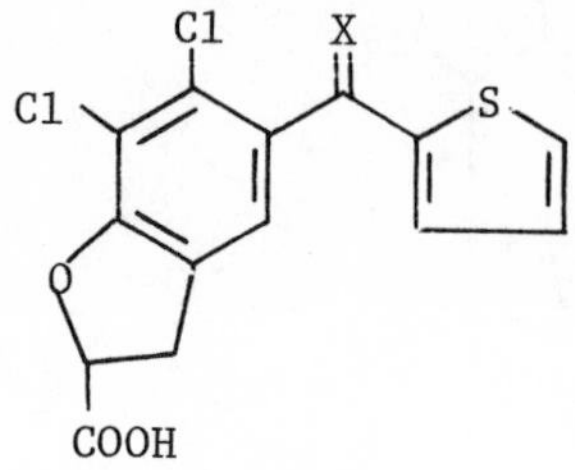

Compd. No.	X	P.O. Biological Activity Scores			
		Diuretic			Uricosuric Chimp
		Rat	Dog	Chimp	
1	O	4	4	4	3
2	H(OH)	1	4*	5*	1
3	H$_2$	±	4	2*	1

*I.V. Data

TABLE XXVI

COLLABORATORS IN THE PHENOXYACETIC ACID RESEARCH

ORGANIC CHEMISTS

A. AUGENBLICK	N.P. GOULD	J.K. HORNER	C.M. ROBB
J.J. BALDWIN	C.N. HABECKER	S.F. KWONG	E.M. SCHULTZ
J.B. BICKING	W.J. HOLTZ	J.W. MASON	J.M. SPRAGUE
W.A. BOLHOFER	W.F. HOFFMAN	F.C. NOVELLO	G.E. STOKKER
A.A. DEANA			T.P. STROBAUGH

PHYSICAL AND ANALYTICAL CHEMISTS

B.H. ARISON	G.V. DOWNING	W.R. MCGAUGHRAN	G.B. SMITH
E.L. CRESSON	Y.C. LEE	W.C. RANDALL	K.B. STREETER

BIOCHEMISTS

D.E. DUGGAN	E.H. HAM	F.A. KUEHL	H.G. OIEN

PHYSICIANS

G.H. BESSELAAR	Z.E. DZIEWANOWSKA	J.J. SCHROGIE	K.F. TEMPERO
R.O. DAVIES			

BIOLOGISTS

J.E. BAER	C.H. DUNCAN	E.K. MAZACK	L.S. WATSON (Dec.)
K.H. BEYER	R.M. EVANS	J.E. MICHAELSON	T.I. WISHOUSKY
D.L. BOHN	G.M. FANELLI	H.F. RUSSO	A.G. ZACCHEI

ACKNOWLEDGMENTS

A. SCRIABINE   R.F. HIRSCHMANN   C.A. STONE

compound 1.

Of the many modifications of the structure of the benzofurans that have been made, one of the more interesting involves
that of the carbonyl group. Reduction to the hydroxymethylene
(one diasteriomer) or to methylene produced compounds which
maintained good activity in dogs and chimpanzees but not in rats
(see Table XXV).

In summary, the rational design of diuretics based upon
either the structural features or mechanism of action of the
mercurial diuretics led to the discovery of about a dozen new
types of potent diuretics. One of these, ethacrynic acid, has
become a clinically useful drug and several others show similar
promise.

We wish to pay tribute to the chemists, biologists and
physicians listed in Table XXVI who contributed to these studies
which were conducted over a period of more than a decade.

Literature Cited

1. Vogl, A., Am. Heart J. (1950), 39, 881.
2. Saxl, P. and Heilig, R., Wien. Klin. Wochschr. (1920),
33, 943.
3. Cafruny, E. J., Pharmacol. Rev. (1968), 20, 89.
4. Schultz, E. M., Cragoe, E. J., Jr., Bicking, J. B.,
Bolhofer, W. A. and Sprague, J. M., J. Med. Pharm. Chem.
(1962), 5, 660.
5. Beyer, K. H., Baer, J. E., Michaelson, J. K. and Russo,
H. F., J. Pharmacol. Exptl. Therap. (1965), 147, 1.
6. Weiner, I. M. and Muller, O. H., ibid. (1955), 113,
241.
7. Zergenyi, J. and Habicht, E., U.S. Patent 3,676,560
(1972).
8. Habicht, E. and Libis, B., U.S. Patent 3,761,494 (1973).
9. Goldberg, M., McCurdy, D. K., Foltz, E. L. and Bluemle,
L. W., Jr., J. Clin. Invest. (1964), 43, 201.
10. Earley, L. E. and Friedler, R. M., ibid. (1964), 43,
1495.
11. Stein, J. H., Wilson, C. B. and Kirkendall, W. M.,
J. Lab. Clin. Med. (1968), 71, 654.
12. Goldberg, M., Am. N. Y. Acad. Sci. (1966), 139, 443.
13. Dirks, J. H., Cirksena, W. J. and Berliner, R. W.,
J. Clin. Invest. (1966), 45, 1875.
14. Kong, Y. H., Arons, G. V., Jr., Dinn, W. M., Jr., Garrison,
G. E. and Orgain, E. S., Circulation (1965), 32, 128.
15. Komorn, R. M. and Cafruny, E. J., Science (1964), 143,
133.
16. Komorn, R. M. and Cafruny, E. J., J. Pharmacol. Exptl.
Therap. (1965), 148, 367.
17. Gussin, R. Z. and Cafruny, E. J., ibid. (1965), 140,
1.
18. Duggan, D. E. and Noll, R. M., Biochim. Biophys. Acta
(1966), 121, 162.

19. Topliss, J. G. and Konzelman, L. M., J. Pharm. Sci. (1968), 57, 737.

20. Bicking, J. B., Robb, C. M., Watson, L. S. and Cragoe, E. J., Jr., ibid. (1976), 544.

21. Bicking, J. B., Holtz, W. J., Watson, L. S. and Cragoe, E. J., Jr., J. Med. Chem. (1976), 19, 530.

22. Schultz, E. M., Bicking, J. B., Deana, A. A., Gould, N. P., Strobaugh, T. P., Watson, L. S. and Cragoe, E. J., Jr., ibid. (1976), 783.

23. Woltersdorf, O. W., Jr., Robb, C. M., Bicking, J. B., Watson, L. S. and Cragoe, E. J., Jr., ibid. (1976), 972.

24. Woltersdorf, O. W., Jr., Cragoe, E. J., Jr., Watson, L. S. and Fanelli, G. M., Jr., 169th Am. Chem. Soc. Mtg., Div. of Med. Chem. Paper No. 48 (1975).

25. Woltersdorf, O. W., Jr., Schneeberg, J. D., Schultz, E. M., Stokker, G. E., Watson, L. S., Fanelli, G. M., Jr. and Cragoe, E. J., Jr., ibid. (1975), Paper No. 49.

26. Cragoe, E. J., Jr., Schultz, E. M., Schneeberg, J. D., Stokker, G. E., Woltersdorf, O. W., Jr., Fanelli, G. M., Jr., Watson, L. S., J. Med. Chem. (1975), 18, 225.

27. Woltersdorf, O. W., Jr., deSolms, S. J., Schultz, E. M. and Cragoe, E. J., Jr., J. Med. Chem. (1977), 20, 1400.

28. deSolms, S. J., Woltersdorf, O. W., Jr., Cragoe, E. J., Jr., Watson, L. S., Fanelli, G. M., Jr., J. Med. Chem. (1978), 21, 437.

29. Cragoe, E. J., Jr. and Woltersdorf, O. W., Jr., U.S. Patent 3,974,212 (1976).

30. Cragoe, E. J., Jr. and Woltersdorf, O. W., Jr., U.S. Patent 4,012,524 (1977).

31. Cragoe, E. J., Jr. and Woltersdorf, O. W., Jr., U.S. Patent 3,976,681 (1976).

32. Watson, L. S., Scriabine, A., Sweet, C. S., Beyer, K. H., Jr., 7th Ann. Am. Soc. Nephr. Mtg. Abst., p. 97 (1974).

33. Watson, L. S., Fanelli, G. M., Russo, H. F., Sweet, C. S., Ludden, C. T. and Scriabine, A. (1976). In New Antihypertensive Drugs, Eds., A. Scriabine and C. S. Sweet, Spectrum Publications, Holliswood, New York.

34. Zacchei, A. G. and Wishousky, T. I., Drug Metab. Dispos. (1976), 4, 490.

35. Zacchei, A. G., Wishousky, T. I., Arison, B. H. and Fanelli, G. M., Jr., Drug Metab. Dispos. (1976), 4, 479.

36. Zacchei, A. G., Wishousky, T. I., Dziewanowska, Z. E., DeSchepper, P. G. and Hitzenberger, G., Europ. J. Metab. Pharmacokin. (1977), 37.

37. Watson, L. S. and Fanelli, G. M., Jr., Fed. Proc. (1975), 34, 802.

38. Fanelli, G. M., Jr., Bohn, D. L., Scriabine, A. and Beyer, K. H., Jr., J. Pharm. Exper. Therap. (1977), 200, 402.

39. Fanelli, G. M., Jr., Bohn, D. L., Zacchei, A. G., J. Pharm. Exper. Therap. (1977), 200, 413.

40. Kauker, M. L., J. Pharm. Exper. Therap. (1977), 200, 81.
41. McKenzie, R., Knight, T. and Weinman, E. J., Proc. Soc.
Exp. Biol.. Med. (1976), 153, 202.
42. Gelarden, R. T. and Beyer, K. H., Jr., Pharmacologist
(1976), 18, 150.
43. Oien, H. G., Babiarz, E. M., Soderman, D. D. and Kuehl, F.
A., Jr., "Prostaglandins in Cardiovascular and Renal Function",
Spectrum Publications, Inc., New York, In Press.
44. Tempero, K. F., Hitzenberger, G., Dziewanowska, Z. E.,
Halkin, H. and Besselaar, G. H., Clin. Pharmacol. & Therap.
(1976), 19, 116.
45. Tempero, K. F., Vedin, J. A., Wilhelmsson, C. E., Lund-
Johansen, P., Vorburger, C., Moerlin, C., Aaberg, H., Enenkel,
W., Bolognese, J. and Dziewanowska, Z. E., Clin. Pharmacol. &
Therap. (1977), 21, 119.
46. Dziewanowska, Z. E., Tempero, K. F., Perret, F.,
Hitenberger, G. and Besselaar, G. H., Clin. Res. (1976), 24,
253A.
47. Cragoe, E. J., Jr. and Woltersdorf, O. W., Jr., U.S. Patent
3,931,239 (1976).
48. Cragoe, E. J., Jr. and Woltersdorf, O. W., Jr., U.S. Patent
3,984,552 (1976).
49. Thuillier, G., Laforest, J., Cariou, B., Bessin, P.,
Bonnet, J. and Thuillier, J., Europ. J. Med. Chim. Therap.
(1974), 9, 625.
50. Cragoe, E. J., Jr. and Woltersdorf, O. W., Jr., U.S. Patent
4,087,542 (1978).

RECEIVED August 21, 1978.

INDEX

INDEX